CW00381145

Rethink Your Diet

Be conscious! And learn how to live a healthy lifestyle.

By: Moein Ghahremani Nejad

Editor: Louise Scrivens

Cover design by: Julya Matsakyan

ISBN-13: 978-1501099267

ISBN-10: 1501099264

To Contact author:

Check the official website of this book:
www.RethinkYourDiet.com

Send a message by email to author: **Moin.ghn@gmail.com**

Connect and send message on official book's page on
Facebook: **www.FaceBook.com/RethinkYourDiet**

MEDICAL DISCLAIMER:
Please note these statements are an account of personal experiences and study. The information and the opinions contained are not intended to diagnose, treat, cure, or prevent any disease.
The statements are in the form of opinions and are not medical evaluations. This material is for information purposes only and is not intended as medical advice. Since there is always some risk involved with publishing alternative health information, the author is not responsible for any adverse effects or consequences resulting from the use of any suggestions or procedures described hereafter. The purpose of publishing this book is to inform readers about the benefits of raw veganism.

Now you can open links easily by using QR codes!
There are many links and URLs in this book, but don't worry, because the author made it easy for you already! For every long link in the book which typing it could be uncomfortable, there is a QR Code which you can use it easily and open the links just by using QR reader on your Smartphone/Tablet.
The QR codes used in this book are usually clustered in a group to use less free space and minimize waste of paper, but there are exactly addressed to prevent from getting confused.
The URL addresses are still there for those individuals who don't have such devices, and also it is necessary for the reader to know the link addresses.
Anyhow, relax and enjoy reading!

Table of Contents

Acknowledgements

I want to offer my gratitude to all the people who helped me to further my knowledge about nutrition and also to write, edit and publish this book.

It's not possible to name them one by one, but I will never forget their help without which this book could not be completed. Their kindness is very much appreciated.

First a special thanks goes to Louise Scrivens for her efforts in editing the book.

Contributions came from many people in many forms including information, research, editing and proofreading.

For their behind-the-scenes contributions, I would like to especially thank Grace Hillis, Ariela Rudy and Jamie Catanese for their kind help in proofreading and thank you to Andrea Lambert for her valuable advice, especially on the subject of cancer.

I would like to thank the authors and publishers who kindly gave me permission to refer to their work to illustrate my points. I have named all of them in my book.

Also my many Iranian friends who have helped me, including Dr. Zarin Azar, and other Iranian raw food authors and activists like Mr. N. Javid and Mr. Houman Naderi, an active raw vegan promoter in Iran. I sincerely thank them all for helping me in such a friendly way.

Finally I would like to add special heartfelt thanks to my parents for all of their support and unconditional love.

Dedication

I dedicate this book to all those who seek true knowledge and consciousness and are willing to change their life to find the answers.

Preface

How content are we with our lives? We must ask ourselves: Is this life worth living?

People are living in hunger, poverty, war and misery throughout the world. Why must so many live through these sufferings? Are these misfortunes and injustices of the world ever going to change?

If we ponder these questions, we will discover that there are bountiful magical sources and gifts this Earth has to offer to mankind, yet we continue to suffer. We are aware that life has existed on Earth for billions of years and has withstood great crises like volcano eruptions, meteor and asteroid strikes, earthquakes and ice ages, and these problems were the major cause of extinction for some living creatures. Nevertheless, life has continued and after each event and massive disaster, life has emerged stronger and more advanced. In other words, Mother Nature uses the worst situations and catastrophes for improvements and we adapt ourselves to them.

How have the cycles of nature been disrupted due to the progression of human civilization?

Undoubtedly, the negative effects of human actions after the Industrial Revolution are very clear, but if we go back further into the past, we will find that diseases, misfortunes, catastrophes and other difficulties were a part of human life well before modern civilization. Even in those days, "wild" and "civilized" people militated together in the worst of ways, destroying nature, life, civilization and anything that crossed their path. Although mankind damaged the environment then, nature was always able to heal itself, making man the victim of his own negative actions.

Unfortunately, following the Industrial Revolution, the human population increased tremendously, resulting in an increase in the devastation of nature. Now, there is no creature on Earth that is safe from mankind's negative actions. However, this is not entirely new or surprising considering the relationship mankind has with itself. Most people don't care about their own behavior or actions amongst themselves, and this applies to the affiliation between men and nature. We can't expect mankind to be kind towards nature and animals when they are making no improvements in their own community. These facts show us that there is an absurdity in human behavior which forces humans to do these unexpected and destructive actions.

Recognizing human faults and taking action to correct them is necessary, which is one reason why we should continue to teach history and other general social lessons to children in school. We must review the past in order to build the future wisely.

Most of our problems in this world, such as environmental destruction and pollution, disease, mental illnesses and social problems are derived from the negative results of improper human development as a result of industrialization and globalization. Due to our wrong decisions, we have achieved a wrong destination which has resulted in wrong actions and has corrupted the human mind. Certainly the so-called "mechanized human" and its related social problems are not an acceptable phenomena, but worse than that the main problems are mechanized contemplation, laziness, egoism, greed, and other inelegances of the human ego that produces subsequent problems and also provokes them.

One must always remember: man is the master of his thoughts and actions. In nature, nothing is harmful by itself until it is used and abused and becomes something it was never meant to be. This is an explicit problem when the very foundation of society has problems itself, therefore, we cannot expect good results if you start with a bad product. We must change the basic building blocks of our thinking and redefine our core values so that they are compatible with new social situations.

It's obvious from the behavior of humans that their mental development is slower in comparison to their handiworks, inventions and artifacts.

The basic idea of civilization is good, but humans don't get ideal results, and industrialization has resulted in poverty, hunger, environmental pollution and insecurity for most people. These problems existed long ago, but now it has grown to the point where thousands are perishing day by day. In addition to this, environmental pollution is killing people and destroying nature. However, just like natural disasters, we could observe that man-made disasters, caused by human actions, are the driving factors of survival in the modern age.

How can we count this foolishness in our daily living as "human's supreme intelligence"? This is not "intelligence", nor is this a "culture". The problems today are clear indications of barbarism - symptoms of inaptitude, foolishness and incapability. The problems humans have created are deep and must be solved at the root cause.

Perhaps you're wondering what these questions and uncertainties about the world have to do with raw veganism and diet. The answer is that human crises are not separate from each other; these issues are closely tied together. In fact, the root of many of our problems is malnutrition, and disease and maladies are only just a few of its negative results.

Our main dilemma in daily life isn't the price of gas, the price of gold, or even the price of smartphones or other expensive possessions. There is something else that needs our attention, something which leads to the death of millions each year, something which causes rampant disease and sickness; it is the food crisis which must take priority over all other concerns.

When there is enough food, no one needs to go after one another; everyone can enjoy the blessings nature has to offer. Only then can we have an ideal civilization and a peaceful life.

It is very clear that I am not the first one to raise such issues. If we take a glance at our past, we see that many great leaders and well-meaning scientists warned us about these problems and even showed us the solutions, yet we as a society barely took heed. However, time is running out and if we don't incorporate these solutions into our daily living, we could become extinct.

It is vital for us to search for efficient solutions and improve them by consulting experts, then choosing the best way to fulfill our daily lives while also correcting the errors of our past. I have applied healthy and sustainable living solutions to my own life with great success.

In this book you will learn about raw veganism and how it can make the world a better place. This book is a compilation of my readings, opinions, experiences, and also comments and suggestions from other experts in this field. My hope and desire is that this book will be a useful guide to all my readers, and I hope that you find the solution to your own personal problems and share the joy with others as well.

My objective

I'm not a medical expert or a scientist, but my curiosity and own health issues led me to ask some very important questions. After my research, I felt that it was my responsibility to find the root of our biggest problems and share my findings with the world.

Many people think that general information means knowing the personal life of Hollywood actors or the political news of the day. Thanks to the technology that we have today, it has paved the way to more useful discoveries. We can use each minute of our life to learn new and useful things. Even more, we can change the way we learn and make more efficient use of our time through Internet research, use online education systems like the Khan Academy[1] or free online courses from universities like MIT or Stanford to further our knowledge. However, whether you put your time towards improving yourself and the world around you or reading useless news, is completely up to you.

This book is my way of continuing the acceleration of public knowledge, helping you learn in a few hundred pages what took me over two years to discover. After you have read this book, you will probably continue to do your own research. If you have suggestions or comments, please share them with me and others.

To make this book more useful, in addition to my research and my experiences, I have included the research of scientists and experts in nutrition, and I have included the citation of the source so you can refer to them directly and do more research on your own. As you know, curiosity is one of the best features of humans, helping us discover something better and something new.

Since the beginning of my veganism journey in October 2011, I have been searching for true and credible information every day, and I have spent a great part of my time reading books, articles, watching documentaries and discussing the issues with other vegans and raw vegans. You can learn everything that I've discovered just by reading this e-book.

One of my readers, a mother-of-four, was diagnosed with heart disease that was so serious that her doctor said that she needed bypass surgery, but she couldn't afford it. After reading my book and trying a raw vegan diet for about three months, she went to the doctor for a checkup and the doctor was amazed at her recovery. She now enjoys a life without any medication. Another positive result of her following the raw vegan diet was that an old eye injury she had suffered for several years became much better, which was very interesting result.

After reading this book, please do not hesitate to send in your comments and suggestions to me via my email address: *Moin.ghn@gmail.com*

Also the book's page on Facebook:
www.FaceBook.com/RethinkYourDiet

If you think this book is helpful, please notify others and help us to play a part in making the world a better place.

With best wishes,
Moein Ghahremani Nejad
September 2014

Chapter 1: Natural Lifestyle and Health

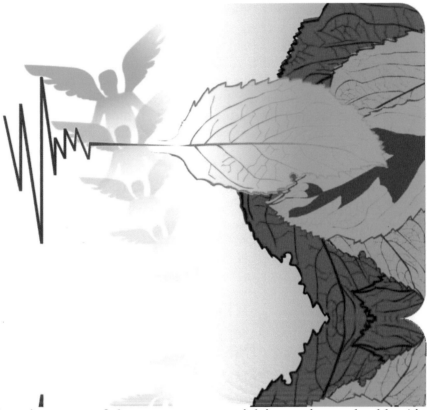

Nowadays, one of the most controversial issues is our health. Air pollution, unhealthy foods, the pressures of work, noise pollution and stress all contribute to causing different diseases and affect the factors that contribute to us recovering from illness.

Even with developments in medical and pharmaceutical sciences, the number of unhealthy people is increasing day by day because many doctors/scientists often don't look at the root causes of illnesses: unhealthy foods, stress and our polluted environment. However doctors try to treat their patients, they can only hide the signs of sickness so after a while the disease returns worse than before. The wretched outcome of this is clear to everyone. Doctors are not to blame here, I am merely pointing out that this medical system is not perfect.

Nearly everyone believes that health is the most valuable gift in life and without it, it's impossible to enjoy other blessings. In other words health isn't everything but without health, everything is nothing.

It is the basic right of every human and every creature to enjoy life, but unfortunately humans have created factors that damage their lives, and not only deprive themselves of a healthy life, but also mar the life of other creatures.

Please note that positive thinking is always helpful. Trying to be positive does not mean that we should ignore the truth. If we don't know the principle of things, we cannot get the results we are looking for, and we only "fall from one pit into a deeper one." (Persian saying)

The first step is identifying the facts and after that, choosing a positive solution to solve the problem. Perhaps the truth is not always what we want to hear, but that doesn't mean we should run from it. As Mahatma Gandhi said: "truth is a bitter medicine which has sweet results."

We know that nowadays it is very rare to find a person who is completely healthy, however many diseases did exist in past centuries but technologies weren't appropriate to detect and cure them, and people lived shorter lives. But on the other hand, some diseases didn't exist at all. In the case of animals they did not suffer the same diseases because they stayed wholly compatible with nature; it was only humans who broke the laws of nature. Unfortunately, nowadays animals on earth also suffer different maladies. This is true especially for pets that are not secure from mankind's harmful actions and artificial life. Nature always went through its intelligent processes without such difficulties, and the problems that did exist, humans only made worse day by day.

In previous decades, open-minded people discovered the secrets of nourishment, and tried their best to spread their findings, but unfortunately most people ignored them because they were lured by the path of money and increasing their gluttony. This tragic destiny is not tolerable anymore.

Now is the time to hear different opinions and choose the option that is most suitable for us. Undoubtedly, different experiences can turn out to be good guides for our lives, and we should learn from the mistakes and achievements of others as well as our own.

This book presents some of the experiments of researchers who looked into our nutrition and health, so that each person can use the findings to make better decisions about their feeding and environmental habits.

Why Raw Veganism?

Research by H. Khorsand on the Body's Self-Healing System

Gholam Hossein Khorsand is an Iranian researcher in nourishment and has treated many patients, including himself, through his food therapy system. I learned a lot about the philosophy of raw eating for the first time from Khorsand's website, which I've been following since March 2011.

Experiences I have referred to from other raw foodists in this book, are for the reader to get a clearer picture. I don't support or reject other methods; I have only used their experiences to make this book more helpful for my readers.

I would like to quote a part of the very interesting philosophy of Khorsand from his website *www.Khorsand.org*. Here is the translated text from Persian to English[2]:

"This philosophy says that all humans and animals need three surviving factors which are held in common: **air**, **water** and **food**. It is necessary to learn about these factors intensely and select the best so we can deliver it to our cells.

Every day new diseases emerge among man while animals do not suffer from illnesses or if they do it is as a result of being in contact with human beings. Animals that live and grow in nature are much healthier than those which are raised by man.

The difference in using the three surviving factors between human beings and animals fall in how we prepare our food: we cook, turn it into useless and toxic material and then eat it which is not practiced by any animal. Apart from that difference, we use the other two factors the same way animals use.

Through some incidents, scientific experiments and continuous studies, I have found out that eating cooked foods which is referred to here as "eating refuse, eating corpse, eating animals" and is widely practiced among intellectual beings, not only isn't necessary but also is a deviation. Similarly, some of us are addicted to smoking, heroin, opium, or alcohol which is wrongly described as a need.

I also discovered that living creatures, including humans, have a vital and sensitive system with a delicate operation which is referred to here as the "body self-healing system". Diseases result from the unawareness of this system and its crucial functions.

The body self-healing system operates around the clock to keep our body clean and protect it from a harmful diet. It segregates all the unwanted elements of food, drink, and air that people have. It feeds the cells with the vital elements, or keeps them for the time that the body doesn't receive efficient food. The system wastes the unwanted elements after the separating process is complete.

Poisons which are released into the bloodstream and partly wasted through kidneys, meet with nerves that make the person feel hungry. The density of the poison causes a severe pain which is similar to the one experienced by the addict. The pain is concealed in the body and its density determines the need of the body for food. A smoker or an addict relieves his pain by smoking and taking drugs, which are not his bodily needs.

The body self-healing system mobilizes cells to collect the old and new wandering poisons in the blood to prevent them from reaching the brain, which can kill the person. (Examples were presented in some of my videos and interviews in which I talked about children who died after eating hamburgers, while their parents, who also ate hamburgers, didn't die. That was because the bodies of the parents produced enough cells throughout the years to get rid of the poisons in the blood. The fake feeling of hunger or the temporary pain disappears for some time while the body is even more contaminated than before).

The old poisons and the new ones are stored in cells and, as a result, disable them. The glands and the organs containing contaminated cells cannot perform their duty as well as they should, and that is when they are wrongly referred to as impaired organs. During medical operations these organs look misshaped and are smelly which mislead professors and proficient surgeons to refer to them as "damaged".

Poisons are stored in the cells because cells are working efficiently! If we eat healthy foods, the blood will be freed from any impurity and can control the poisons; therefore, the cells can release the poisons into the bloodstream and return to their original functions. Consequently, there will be no impaired organs and the body functions normally.

The process explained above reoccurs (in a more painful way) after a few hours and when the body self-healing system completes the process of analyzing new foods to separate and waste the poisons, which are denser and more life-threatening and enter the body through cooked food, medicines, smoking, drugs and so on.

Once more the body healing system commands the cells to gather up the impurities. In dealing with the impurities, the cells (that are wrongly considered microbes and the cause of pains; misleadingly called sicknesses) function in different ways. These cells are all in the body and are well prepared to take care of the unwanted elements.

Unknowingness about how the body self-healing system works results in harmful actions.

The more cooked foods you eat and the more medicines you take, the more cells will be overwhelmed with stored poisons; therefore the body becomes more contaminated. Pains diverge and the number of cells, glands and organs whose functionality reduce or halt, increase. As the pains vary, the poisons will form new shapes. At this point, more cells are occupied, there are fewer active and healthy cells to refine the blood, and no medicine will heal the pains.

This is the main cause of diseases that could not be cured despite the fact that thousands of research intuitions have discovered millions of medicines so far. Diseases diverge and increase. The body self-healing system remains unaware. Newly discovered medicines are in vain; this cycle goes on and thousands of individuals lose their lives.

The whole painful process could be prevented simply by converting to a vegetarian diet. The body would get cleaned and those complicated pains and diseases foreclosed, and cells would not store poisons. The treatment can start by eating vegetables and uncooked foods which cure weaknesses, make cells function healthy and get rid of the unwanted elements efficiently and effectively.

This treatment has seen positive outcomes throughout the years; anecdotes by treated patients prove it. The most productive treatment is being vegetarian and avoiding eating cooked foods either temporarily or permanently.

You might have more or less experienced this with loved ones who have passed due to a simple illness. They took medicines hoping they would feel better but this did not happen, the disease became complicated and various medications were prescribed. The medicines cured the disease temporarily, no sound treatment took place, and more cells became damaged until there was no healthy cell left in the body. As a result they died because their cells were full of poisons. If anyone turns to vegetarianism (raw-eating) for treatment after undergoing a long conventional medication process and there was no positive result, be sure that no other treatment could help that person. His corrupt cells could not be replaced in any other way, too."

Khorsand's theory on what cooked foods do to our bodies are based on his experiments on the adroit pigeons and also references to raw food eating in ancient ages from a poem in "Shahnameh"; a historic book of poems written by Ferdowsi, the famous Persian poet around ten centuries ago.

The Pigeon's experience[3]

Khorsand recalls: "A memory from my childhood that has always stuck with me and has since saved me from sickness and death and hopefully it will also save the world from sickness and ignorance.

We had a relatively large house in Khorramshar, Iran - which was made in the old customary style of its time with a yard all around the house and six large rooms laid out in a way that the northern side had five entrance doors and before that was a high porch. On the eastern and western sides it had three large basements where in the hot weather of Khorramshar city, we used to use them to get together and enjoy parties.

This house had an old-fashioned traditional and amazing design.

It had nice air conditioning and in the middle of the back yard there was a tall palm tree that used to give us a lot of dates and even now tens of years later I can still taste those dates in my mouth! Because for as long as I can remember I used to spend a lot of time up that tree when I was a child. It was a place that I could see all the surrounding areas.

In this large traditional house with lots of good memories, my brother had lots of pigeons, 30 or 40.

Apparently these pigeons were very special pigeons because they were so healthy and fit that they used to fly for long hours (as much as eight hours) in the sky above our house and they used to fly so high at times that they would disappear. My brother and his friends used to watch these pigeons from the roof of the house and he used to brag about their performance calling each one of those pigeons by their special name.

Maybe I was eight or nine years old when one day we were sitting in the backyard with the rest of the family enjoying a picnic. We were eating lunch and my big brother, Bijan, who was fourteen years old, before eating, he would take a large white bag that had wheat, grains, seeds or raw lentils and would throw a handful of it on to the other side of the yard far enough so that the pigeons could feed themselves and at the same time he would keep them away from us so we could have our lunch. This way he would then sit next to me so he could have his lunch.

It wasn't long before the pigeons would finish all the raw seeds and they would come close to us again and in order for me to keep the pigeons away from us and give Bijan a little extra time to eat his lunch, I would throw a handful of my cooked rice for them.

I would throw a few spoons of the rice that I was eating in the farthest part of the yard and in the beginning you would see that the pigeons would run towards the rice that I had thrown but they quickly returned and the cooked rice would remain untouched.

This caused my three brothers and two sisters to laugh at me and say: "now you have to go and clean up all the rice you've thrown there".

The pigeons rejecting the rice that us humans had eaten amazed me and it was hard for me to believe.

I was asking myself if there were hidden secrets and reasons behind their actions that we humans were unaware of.

But quickly I remembered that there were plenty of chickens which I had seen eating bread and the rice and I would say to myself that maybe it was because, despite having wings, they can't fly like my brother's pigeons.

Because of my curiosity about this disliking of the rice by the pigeons, an idea came to me.

After my brother and the rest of my family returned to their rooms I returned to the backyard with the reason of cleaning up the rice which the pigeons didn't eat and then with a quick attack I was able to catch two of the pigeons and take them to one of the basements in my house. There I found a large square metal pail which was about one meter by one meter and I used it as a cage and I imprisoned the pigeons inside this cage that I had found and I put the open end of this cage against the wall so that the pigeons could not run away. I put a little bit of water for them in this box that had now became a house for these two poor pigeons and I remember telling them that if they wanted to be stubborn (by rejecting the food I'd thrown for them) I was more stubborn than them and I would keep them like this until they had eaten the rice as we humans did!

A few hours passed by and I returned to the basement to check on the pigeons and from the few holes in the pail I noticed they were sitting in a corner of the box far away from the rice and they had not eaten anything.

Anyway after checking on them a few more times I realized that the poor pigeons, against their own will and because of their hunger, had broken their food strike and were starting to eat some of the rice.

I repeated the same thing for about 14 days and I would put out the same rice and water for them. Fortunately my brother, after searching for these two pigeons, concluded that they had flown far away and he would say that they would return after a few days as had happened with previous pigeons.

After a few weeks on an occasion when Bijan was not in the house, I took out the two prisoners from this metal box to see if anything had changed. The first thing I noticed was these pigeons had gotten extremely fat but the fatness was in a bad way. They looked really out of shape. I saw that they had developed large breasts. I took them outside in the backyard and released them and noticed that just as a new chick which had just hatched, they would carry their chests very close to the ground and they couldn't stand on their feet very well. They couldn't avoid dragging their breasts on the ground. I think they didn't have any energy in their feet and generally they were shaking and looking very sick.

As an experiment I took one of them and I wanted to make it fly but that poor pigeon was like a stone and without even shaking its wings, fell down on the ground on its face.

This was a very strange incident.

What did this cooked rice do to them?! In the neighborhood there was an old couple that lived there and the kids in the neighborhood used to call them Aa-baba and Bibi or grandpa and grandma, and they used to always call me to do something for them, for example, help them to cross rivulet or high lands.

I compared them to these birds and thought because they ate a lot of cooked rice, now they had become so weak that they had to walk with canes and they didn't see well.

I started to think that in the cooked rice and in the cooked food there may be some molecules that cause the human body to decay and make us disabled and sick over time.

Also in Shahnameh (the ancient Persian book about the history of Persia) it is mentioned clearly that in previous centuries in Persia, people were eating only fruits and vegetables and they didn't kill animals for food, but a great deviancy occurred so then they fell into adversity."

Treating damaged kidneys leads to a great discovery

Here I translated a Persian interview with Mr. H. Khorsand on his website in which he explains his personal experiment with raw eating.

People want to know about your experiment which is the cause of your philosophy.

H. Khorsand: "Yes, and I think this is very necessary for others to know about the basis of my philosophy.

As for my experiment in my childhood (the story of pigeons which is explained in the previous pages of this book) and after seeing the fatigue in old men and women and the different diseases people suffer, I found a connection between these phenomena and my experiment with the pigeons, and a great doubt initiated in me about the nourishing of humankind and it forced me to do more research, until unfortunately (or perhaps, fortunately) I myself became a patient when I suffered kidney damage. One of my kidneys was sick and I started treatment only to find both of them became sick! All the doctors I saw in KhorramShahr City, Tehran and England said that my kidneys were corrupted and they should remove my kidneys immediately; this was after many checkups and using many medicines.

When I wanted to go to Tehran for treatment, my friends and family weren't optimistic about it because the doctors said that it was possible at any second that my kidneys could stop completely and I would die immediately! And I believed this.

My only hope was going to one of the best hospitals in the world in London so my doctor in Tehran got a recommendation for me to go there for treatment.

In London, after many checkups and radiology, they confirmed the statements of my doctors in Iran and said that my left kidney should be removed immediately.

For me there was no other way when I was bedridden in a famous hospital in London, but I wanted to at least survive after this tormenting surgery during my youth. This wasn't a big expectation! And at least, I thought, this surgery would help my other kidney so it could perform its duty. But unfortunately this medical science couldn't guarantee this even for me as a young man! They couldn't even guarantee my survival!

They wanted me to decide within 48 hours whether I wanted my kidney removed, because they were very busy.

I had come to London with many wishes, but unfortunately even in this [developed country], there wasn't any good news.

I was musing in sadness and I saw my efforts in the past like a movie in front of my eyes. I imagined the face of my friends and family and asked myself: "Will I see them again?!" and also I asked myself like a mad man: "Why?! Why did I catch this big torture in my youth?" and I regretted it because there was no solution for me, and any real treatment should treat my kidneys not cut them out!

My God! So what I should do?

I thought back to my childhood…. suddenly, I remembered my experiment with pigeons, and my mind was attracted to a philosophy which was initiated inside me, and less than 24 hours before the determined deadline, I decided to test my philosophy. I refused to have surgery and instead left the hospital feeling powerful.

I changed my nourishment and controlled it strongly, and as a result, my kidneys were treated in less than three months with small amounts of date palm, walnut and other gifts from God, whereas all doctors and medicines not only couldn't treat me, but also made my condition worse to the point where I faced the possibility of death.

Now more than fifty years later, my kidneys are wholly healthy, and I was lucky that I didn't follow dictations from doctors and I didn't give up and I didn't let them get my money and mutilate me respectfully! If not, I would have died many years ago.

After that, I shared my experiences with others and I could treat many patients with my natural method."

The enzymes in raw foods: a debatable theory

The enzyme theory is a popular theory between some raw foodists, however it is a debatable theory as well. This theory claims that many useful enzymes and co-enzymes in raw foods are destroyed after being heated to more than 46 degrees centigrade. All cooked foods are divested from enzymes so the body is compelled to sprinkle more enzymes to digest the foods, and it causes the body's glands and organs to wear out in a short time.

Some experts believe that enzymes in living foods are very important. This has been illustrated through research carried out by scientists such as Artturi Ilmari Virtanen, a Finnish chemist and recipient of the 1945 Nobel Prize in chemistry. He showed that enzymes in raw foods which are destroyed by cooking and baking, are very important in aiding digestion. They also help aid the absorbency of foods with less pressure on the body. But when enzymes in natural foods are destroyed by cooking, it becomes harder to digest and absorb foods and the body reacts by discharging more enzymes causing our bodies to tire quicker.

On the other hand, some experts, even some raw vegan pioneers, do not believe in this enzyme theory, and most of them suggest very logical reasons to justify this. For example Dr. Douglas Graham, who is a raw vegan pioneer and is famous for the "80/10/10" diet, explains:

"Enzymes function as the organic chemistry version of catalysts, meaning that they facilitate chemical reactions but do not get involved in the reaction, coming out of it unchanged. A lot of hype has been created around enzymes, misinformation that has really caught on within the raw food movement. A few facts are in order. Our body produces the enzymes it needs to make digestion happen. There are some 20 different enzymes responsible for the digestion of proteins, fats, and carbohydrates. If the digestive enzymes we required to digest foods were already within the foods, the foods would digest themselves.[4]"

Another explanation which can increase our knowledge in this area is an explanation by Dr. Joel Fuhrman, a vegan pioneer who believes in the benefits of low-temperature cooking and promotes one of the healthiest diets around. He writes:

"It is true that when food is baked at high temperatures—and especially when it is fried or barbecued—toxic compounds are formed and important nutrients are lost. Many vitamins are water-soluble, and a significant percent can be lost with cooking, especially overcooking. Similarly, many plant enzymes function as phytochemical nutrients in our body and can be useful to maximize health. They, too, can be destroyed by overcooking.

Enzymes are proteins that work to speed up or "catalyze" chemical reactions. Every living cell makes enzymes for its own activities. Human cells are no exception. Our glands secrete enzymes into the digestive tract to aid in the digestion of food. However, after they are ingested, the enzymes contained in plants do not function as enhancements or replacements for human digestive enzymes. These molecules exist to serve the plant's purpose, not ours. The plant enzymes get digested by our own digestive juices along with the rest of the food and are absorbed and utilized as nutrients.

Contrary to what many raw-food web sites claim, the enzymes contained in the plants we eat do not catalyze chemical reactions that occur in humans. The plant enzymes merely are broken down into simpler molecules by our own powerful digestive juices. Even when the food is consumed raw, plant enzymes do not aid in their own digestion inside the human body. It is not true that eating raw food demands less enzyme production by your body, and dietary enzymes inactivated by cooking have an insignificant effect on your health and your body's enzymes.[5]"

By following a raw vegan diet we become healthier, feel better and more energized. The main reason is not only enzymes, but also because raw foods are easier to digest by our body, as will explain further as we go on.

There is no doubt that humans denature foods by cooking them at high temperatures making them harder to digest.

On the basis of different experiences and also other scientific evidence, even if we don't believe in one particular theory we will find that raw foodism (meaning that at least 80% of our diet is based on raw plant foods) is much better than unhealthy traditional or modern diets.

The importance of eating raw food

In the past, some scientists have attempted to produce food pills taking away the need to eat fresh food but fortunately these attempts failed for many reasons, one of which was the inability to reproduce the mineral and nutrient content that fresh foods provide in a pill.

The minerals in soil aren't useful for animals but plants use these minerals and turn them into organic (living) matter that can be useful for animals' body cells. A calcium pill isn't the same as the living calcium found in plants, because to make it possible for the body to absorb calcium, it needs other nutrients such as vitamin D, magnesium and vitamin A.

If we were to eat one calcium pill, one vitamin D pill, one vitamin A pill and others to help our body to absorb calcium, this would be ineffective because there are many other foodstuffs found in fresh organic foods as well as calcium which our bodies need.

Sometimes, some animals like elephants[6] and parrots[7] eat soil because they are lacking certain minerals and nutrients but their main requirement is live foods to remain healthy.

These minerals and nutrients along with biotic materials such as oxygen found in live foods are destroyed when we cook food. Raw natural foods contain a little oxygen which is destroyed during the cooking process. This oxygen is maybe necessary for chemical reactions during digestion. In addition to this most cooked foods are heavy to digest, so they waste the oxygen and enzymes inside our body to digest them. To oxygenate the body it needs a balanced plant-based diet.[8]

Water is vital for our body and helps with our everyday detoxification but the pure water found in fresh plants evaporates when we cook it. What is important to note is the pipes which carry water to our homes is full of chlorine, polluted with microscopic fungus and can often be corroded so we cannot compare this water to natural water found in fresh foods. It is better to be a raw-eater so we can fully benefit from this natural water and opt for a good water purification machine to provide the rest of our daily water needs.

Raw foods are already cooked by nature

To describe foods as raw or living doesn't mean they are unprepared. Natural foods are cooked by the sun during the photosynthesis process.

Crude soil is turned into natural foods by plants, but when we cook natural foods, we kill them and turn them into non-organic mineral matter. By heating food at high temperatures, all the vital energy of food is destroyed along with its vitamins and proteins. If you plant a cooked bean in the soil it will not grow, while raw beans will always grow.

If we think natural live foods are not delicious and we should destroy them by cooking, this is because:

#1. We have grown accustomed to cooking and it is has changed our palate.

#2. We consume foods which as humans are not our natural foods, so they don't seem tasty to us at first.

When we start changing our diet to what it should be naturally, we will soon become accustomed and our taste buds will change, especially if we increase fruits and vegetables in our diet. Even if we start by incorporating just a little of these foods into our diet which we're not used to eating, such as grains in their sprouted state, we will soon enjoy the taste and health benefits.

 To eat food which is not compatible with our digestive system is a problem, but cooking that food usually makes it even worse, for example grains, beans and all animal foods become more harmful when cooked. Those who have followed a raw food diet from a young age often don't like the taste of cooked foods at all showing what our natural diet should be.

The physiological reasons for being a vegan[9]

There are many reasons which show humans are meant to be vegan. Some obvious reasons are:

#1: Teeth, tongue, jaws and nails + running speed

Teeth: Humans have short, soft fingernails and pathetically small canine teeth. In contrast, carnivores all have sharp claws and large canine teeth capable of tearing flesh.

The molars of a carnivore are pointed and sharp. Ours are primarily flat, for mashing food. Our "canine" teeth bear no resemblance to true fangs. Nor do we have a mouthful of them, as a true carnivore does.

Dental Formula: Mammalogists use a system called the "dental formula" to describe the arrangement of teeth in each quadrant of the jaws of an animal's mouth. This refers to the number of incisors, canines, and molars in each of the four quadrants. Starting from the center and moving outward, our formula, and that of most anthropoids, is 2/1/5. The dental formula for carnivores is 3/1/5-to-8.

Tongues: Only the truly carnivorous animals have rasping (rough) tongues. All other creatures have smooth tongues.

Carnivores' jaws move only up and down, requiring them to tear chunks of flesh off their prey and swallow them whole. Humans and other herbivores can move their jaws up and down and from side to side, allowing them to grind up fruit and vegetables with their back teeth. Like other herbivores' teeth, human back molars are flat for grinding fibrous plant foods. Carnivores lack these flat molars.

Dr. Richard Leakey, a renowned anthropologist, summarizes: "You can't tear flesh by hand, you can't tear hide by hand. Our anterior teeth are not suited for tearing flesh or hide. We don't have large canine teeth, and we wouldn't have been able to deal with food sources that require those large canines."

Although there are different views about canine teeth and some people believe that our teeth are for meat-eating, it seems that's not true at all because fruitarian monkeys also have the same canine teeth which are much bigger than ours, but they are vegetarian.

Carnivores run very fast and they can hunt while running and get their victim using their mouth, but humans can't. Instead, humans can take vegetables from the earth and climb trees and gather fruits easily.

There are other reasons which prove that humans were meant to be pure vegetarians (or more precisely frugivores) and after reading them, it's very reasonable to say humans were actually meant to be vegan as we're most similar to other plant-eaters, and drastically different from carnivores and true omnivores[10].

#2: Stomach Acidity

Carnivores swallow their food whole, relying on their extremely acidic stomach juices to break down flesh and kill the dangerous bacteria in meat that would otherwise sicken or kill them. The concentration of the stomach acid of carnivores is several times stronger than that of herbivores and humans. Our stomach acid is much weaker in comparison because a strong acid is not needed to digest pre-chewed fruits and vegetables. So meat alone isn't a complete food for humans at all and it's impossible for humans to eat the bones of animals in their natural state.

#3: Intestinal length

Carnivores have short intestinal tracts and colons that allow meat to pass through them relatively quickly, before it can rot and cause illness. Humans' intestinal tracts are much longer than those of carnivores of a comparable size. Longer intestines allow the body more time to break down fiber and absorb the nutrients from plant-based foods, but they make it dangerous for humans to eat meat. The bacteria in meat have extra time to multiply during the long trip through the digestive system, increasing the risk of food poisoning. Meat actually begins to rot while it makes its way through human intestines, which increases the risk of colon cancer.

Eating meat disarranges the proceeds of useful bacteria in the human intestine. It is estimated that there are millions of bacteria living in the human intestine. Most of these microscopic creatures are useful bacteria but it seems that they can't remain useful when combined with toxins from meat. The poisons kill many useful bacteria and also many of these useful bacteria become harmful because of their dangerous excrement after using toxins. But this doesn't happen with vegetables and fruits and in fact, better digestion and absorption of vital nutrients is accomplished with the controlled yeast of useful bacteria.

#4: Sleep

Humans spend roughly two thirds of every 24-hour cycle actively awake. Carnivores typically sleep and rest from 18 to 20 hours per day and sometimes more.

#5: Vision

Our sense of vision responds to the full spectrum of color, making it possible to distinguish ripe from unripe fruit at a distance.
Meat eaters do not typically see in full color.

#6: Meal Size

Fruit is in scale to our food requirements. It fits our hands. A few pieces of fruit is enough to make a meal, leaving no waste.
Carnivores typically eat the entire animal when they kill it which would normally be too much food for one person's meal.

#7: Human Psychology

Humans also lack the instinct that drives carnivores to kill animals and devour their raw carcasses. While carnivores take pleasure in killing animals and eating their raw flesh, any human who killed an animal with his or her bare hands and ate the raw corpse would be considered deranged. Carnivorous animals are excited by the scent of blood and the thrill of the chase. Most humans, on the other hand, are revolted by the sight of blood, intestines and raw flesh, and cannot tolerate hearing the screams of animals being ripped apart and killed. The bloody reality of eating animals is innately repulsive to us; another indication that we were not designed to eat meat.

#8: If we were meant to eat meat, why is it killing us?

Carnivorous animals in the wild virtually never suffer from heart disease, cancer, diabetes, strokes, or obesity; ailments that appear in humans largely due to the consumption of saturated fat and cholesterol in meat.

#9: Fat and cholesterol

Studies have shown that even when fed 200 times the amount of animal fat and cholesterol that the average human consumes each day, carnivores do not develop the hardening of the arteries that leads to heart disease and strokes in humans.

Researchers have actually found that it is impossible for carnivores to develop hardening of the arteries, no matter how much animal fat they consume.

On the other hand humans were not designed to process animal flesh, so all the excess fat and cholesterol from a meat-based diet makes us sick. Heart disease, for example, is the number one killer in America according to the American Heart Association, and medical experts agree that this ailment is largely the result of consuming animal products.

Meat eaters have a 50 percent higher risk of developing heart disease than vegetarians.

#10: Food Poisoning

Since we don't have strong stomach acid like carnivores to kill all the bacteria in meat, dining on animal flesh can also give us food poisoning. According to the USDA, meat is the cause of 70 percent of food borne illnesses in the United States because it's often contaminated with dangerous bacteria like E.coli, Listeria, and Campylobacter. Every year in the United States alone, food poisoning sickens over 75 million people and kills more than 5,000.

Dr. William C. Roberts, M.D., editor of the authoritative *American Journal of Cardiology* sums it up this way: "although we think we are one and we act as if we are one, human beings are not natural carnivores. When we kill animals to eat them, they end up killing us because their flesh, which contains cholesterol and saturated fat, was never intended for human beings, who are natural herbivores."

#11: Excessive protein in meat and eggs + the dangers of other animal's milk for the body

We consume twice as much protein as we need when we eat a meat-based diet, and this contributes to osteoporosis and kidney stones. Animal protein raises the acid level in our blood, causing calcium to be excreted from the bones to restore the blood's natural pH balance. This calcium depletion leads to osteoporosis, and the excreted calcium ends up in the kidneys, where it can form kidney stones or even trigger kidney disease.

Consuming animal protein has also been linked to cancer of the colon, breast, prostate, and pancreas. According to Dr. T. Colin Campbell, the director of the Cornell-China-Oxford Project on Nutrition[11], Health, and the Environment: "in the next ten years, one of the things you're bound to hear is that animal protein is one of the most toxic nutrients of all that can be considered."

Egg and dairy also have the same negative effect on the human body. Each egg has almost 10 times more protein than the human body needs (per day) so it damages the liver and kidneys and dairy also makes human blood acidic and in nature, we know it's very rare that a mammal consumes the milk of another mammal. Many researchers have found that only its mother's milk is the best milk for babies and many moral and adventitious features are transferred to babies from the milk which he drinks, so milk from one animal isn't good for another animal. Cow's milk (and also other animals' milk) is very different from human milk as it has much more protein, minerals and fat than human milk because it's supposed to be food for calves, not us.

Milk sugar is not good for adults, so even a human mother's milk isn't useful and enough for adults. Thus, we can easily understand why the milk of other animals isn't suitable for adults at all. It seems that milk can have negative effects on diabetes and different cancers and it will cause many problems in the intestines and derange digestion. Homogenized milk, in particular, is very harmful. Also if we dilute milk with water, protein and fats from the milk it can't break up properly in the water so what is produced is a non-equal mixture which causes different digestive problems. Remember that in nature it's very rare that a baby animal drinks the milk of another species. Perhaps it occasionally takes place, but only for cubs and babies, not for adults.

There are also the negative effects of different antibiotics and stress on animals whose meat and milk we consume. These make animal products more and more dangerous.

Eating meat can also have negative consequences for stamina and sexual potency. One Danish study indicated that: "men peddling on a stationary bicycle until muscle failure lasted an average of 114 minutes on a mixed meat and vegetable diet, 57 minutes on a high-meat diet, and a whopping 167 minutes on a strict vegetarian diet." Besides having increased physical endurance, vegan men are also less likely to suffer from impotence.

#12: Our saliva

Our saliva contains Alpha-Amylase, an enzyme that digests plant foods, which is not found in the saliva of carnivores.

#13: Saliva and Urine PH

All of the plant-eating creatures (including healthy humans) maintain alkaline saliva and urine most of the time.
However, the saliva and urine of the meat eating animals is acidic.

#14: Diet pH

Carnivores thrive on a diet of acid-forming foods; such a diet is deadly for humans, setting the stage for a wide variety of diseases. Our preferred foods are all alkaline-forming.

#15: Stomach acid pH

The level of the hydrochloric acid that humans produce in their stomachs generally ranges about 3 to 4 or higher but can go as low as 2.0. (0 being most acidic, 7 neutral and 14 most alkaline).

The stomach acid of cats and other meat eaters can be in the 1^+ range and usually runs in the 2s. Because the pH scale is logarithmic this means the stomach acid of a carnivore is at least 10 times stronger than that of a human and can be 100 or even 1,000 times stronger.

#16: Digestive Enzymes

Our digestive enzymes are geared to easily digest fruit. We produce ptyalin, also known as salivary amylase, to initiate the digestion of fruit. Meat-eating animals do not produce any ptyalin and have completely different digestive enzyme ratios.

#17: Sugar Metabolism

The glucose and fructose in fruits fuel our cells without straining our pancreas (unless we eat a high-fat diet). Meat eaters do not handle sugars well. They are prone to diabetes if they eat a diet that is predominated by sugar.

#18: Intestinal flora

Humans have different bacterial colonies (flora) living in their intestines than those found in carnivorous animals. The ones that are similar, such as lactobacillus and E.coli are found in different ratios in the plant eaters' intestines compared to those of the carnivores.

#19: Cleanliness

We are the most particular of all creatures about the cleanliness of our food. Carnivores are the least picky, and will eat dirt, bugs, organic debris, and other items along with their food.

#20: Drinking water and perspiring

Carnivores lap up water and plants to get rid of body heat. Humans sip water and perspire through pores in the skin.

#21: Mouth size

Carnivores' mouths are very big, so that they can hold a big part of another animal, enabling them to hunt.

The human mouth is small and it can't be used for hunting other animals at all. Thus, this is another reason which shows humans are vegetarian.

#22: Olfaction

Carnivores can inhale and feel the scent of other animals from a great distance, but humans don't have this ability.

#23: Our reaction to carnivores

Herbivorous animals recognize their kind very well; for example, hens move under cows and search for food without any fear, but if a wolf or fox comes close to them, they flee immediately. Humans also flee from carnivores too.

#24: Spiritual consciousness

Food is the source of the body's chemistry, and what we ingest affects our consciousness, emotions and experiential pattern. If we want to live in a higher consciousness, feeling peace and happiness and love for all creatures, then we should consider not eating meat, fish, shellfish, fowl, eggs or milk.

An analogy table for comparing Carnivores, Omnivores and Humans Meat contains absolutely nothing - no proteins, vitamins or minerals - that the human body cannot obtain perfectly well from a vegetarian diet.

Milton R. Mills, M.D. wrote an excellent paper which covers the anatomy of eating[12] , so I've included it in brief that summarizes his research which clearly shows that humans are biologically herbivores:

Facial muscles

Carnivores: Reduced to allow wide mouth gape
Omnivores: Reduced
Herbivores: Well-developed
Humans: Well-developed

Jaw type

Carnivores: Angle not expanded
Omnivores: Angle not expanded
Herbivores: Expanded angle
Humans: Expanded angle

Jaw joint location

Carnivores: On same plane as molar teeth
Omnivores: On same plane as molar teeth
Herbivores: Above the plane of the molars
Humans: Above the plane of the molars

Jaw motion

Carnivores: Shearing; minimal side-to-side motion
Omnivores: Shearing; minimal side-to-side motion
Herbivores: No shear; good side-to-side, front-to-back
Humans: No shear; good side-to-side, front-to-back

Major jaw muscles

Carnivores: Temporalis
Omnivores: Temporalis
Herbivores: Temporalis
Humans: Masseter and pterygoids

Mouth opening vs. head size

Carnivores: Large
Omnivores: Large
Herbivores: Small
Humans: Small

Teeth: Incisors

Carnivores: Short and pointed
Omnivores: Short and pointed
Herbivores: Broad, flattened and spade-shaped
Humans: Broad, flattened and spade-shaped

Teeth: Canines
Carnivores: Long, sharp and curved
Omnivores: Long, sharp and curved
Herbivores: Dull and short or long (for defense), or none
Humans: Short and blunted

Teeth: Molars
Carnivores: Sharp, jagged and blade-shaped
Omnivores: Sharp blades and/or flattened
Herbivores: Flattened with cusps vs. complex surface
Humans: Flattened with nodular cusps

Chewing
Carnivores: None; swallows food whole
Omnivores: Swallows food whole and/or simple crushing
Herbivores: Extensive chewing necessary
Humans: Extensive chewing necessary

Saliva
Carnivores: No digestive enzymes
Omnivores: No digestive enzymes
Herbivores: Carbohydrate digesting enzymes
Humans: Carbohydrate digesting enzymes

Stomach acidity with food in stomach
Carnivores: $\leq$ pH 1
Omnivores: $\leq$ pH 1
Herbivores: pH 4-5
Humans: pH 4-5

Length of small intestine
Carnivores: 3-6 times body length
Omnivores: 4-6 times body length
Herbivores: 10-12+ times body length
Humans: 10-11 times body length

Colon
Carnivores: Simple, short, and smooth
Omnivores: Simple, short, and smooth
Herbivores: Long, complex; may be sacculated

Humans: Long, sacculated

Liver
Carnivores: Can detoxify vitamin A
Omnivores: Can detoxify vitamin A
Herbivores: Cannot detoxify vitamin A
Humans: Cannot detoxify vitamin A

Kidney
Carnivores: Extremely concentrated urine
Omnivores: Extremely concentrated urine
Herbivores: Moderately concentrated urine
Humans: Moderately concentrated urine

Nails
Carnivores: Sharp claws
Omnivores: Sharp claws
Herbivores: Flattened nails or blunt hooves
Humans: Flattened nails

The details are in Mills' paper[13].

Comparing the human body with other animals

#1. We sleep about the same amount of time as other herbivores, and less than carnivores and true omnivores.

#2. Omnivore doesn't mean to eat 50% plants and 50% animals. Many consider chimpanzees to be omnivores but 95-99% of their diet is plants, and most of the rest isn't meat, it is termites. If humans are omnivores, then the anatomical evidence suggests that we're the same kind - the kind that eats almost exclusively plant foods.

#3. Even the eyes of carnivores are different from herbivores, and they can see in the dark while humans can't.

#4. It's very difficult to eat raw meat because it's very rigid and we can't chew it like carnivores can.

#5. Pregnant women usually desire more fruits and vegetables during their pregnancy, because their babies need these natural foods for growth.

How to learn from animals
In the book "Raw Secrets" by Frederic Patenaude[14], he refers to a study by Albert Mosséri[15] which is very noteworthy:

Mosséri quotes another natural hygienist:
"During the years I spent in Central America and in Cuba, I had the opportunity to observe the
reaction of monkeys when offered a food they had never eaten before. Instinctively, they use three senses to tell if the food is poisonous:
• The sense of sight
• The sense of smell
• The sense of taste
First they attentively look at the new food. If it passes this first exam of the sense of sight, they

35

pursue their examination with their acute sense of smell. They bring their nose close to this new food and smell it intensely. If they find it has a pleasant smell, it will have passed this part of the inspection. Finally, they lick the food and taste a small piece of it. If they like the taste, they start to eat it carefully.

During this whole process, the animal has acted according to the Universal Law of Natural Dietetics; that is, they found the new food to be:

• Pleasant to the sight
• Pleasant to the smell
• Pleasant to the taste

When it was consumed:

• In the raw state
• Without combinations
• Without seasonings

This law is known by all animals, who obey it… all except man.

Theofilio de la Torre
As quoted by Mosséri in La Nourriture Idéale

To this information from Torre, a natural hygienist of the 19th Century, let us add that through the process of civilization, we humans have lost much of our instinct. We cannot rely on it entirely (the mistake of "instinctive eating"). Everyone, more or less, has a debased instinct. For this reason, many authors observed children in order to get clues on what should be our natural diet."

The differences between the diet of apes and the diet of humans

Let us now look at the diet of apes and gorillas, which are said to be closely related to humans.

Even chimps sometimes eat fish, but first, they always eat fish in its natural raw state and they savor its taste. Secondly they usually eat fish with their bare hands, without any tools, while humans instinctively use tools to eat. Thirdly these foods (like fish and insects) make up only a small part of a chimp's diet (1% or less).

Chimps sometimes even eat each other. However, this doesn't necessarily mean that they need animal food it may be that they are adapting to tough environmental situations such as when there is a lack of foods. Despite this their anatomy isn't designed for eating meat, because their bodies are similar to herbivores.

In addition, if we compare chimps with gorillas, we will see that gorillas usually eat fruit and greens and only sometimes eat insects, not fish or other animal products, but the gorilla is bigger and more powerful than chimps.

I have been interested in this subject for a while, and recall the opinion of a person who disagreed with veganism who told me: "when monkeys eat insects, this shows that the body needs animal protein. We humans are similar to them, so we should eat animal protein, too." However, I believe if they eat insects for the sake of animal protein, they should eat more insects regularly, not sometimes and only about 1% of their total diet.

We know that every animal in nature gets its required protein needs from what it eats frequently, not what it eats occasionally. Therefore, perhaps this action of monkeys has another reason that we don't know yet. For example it could be because of useful bacteria in the body of insects.

The human body has many differences to a gorilla's body; for example there are more starch digestive enzymes (amylase) in human saliva than in the human digestive system, several times more than monkeys. The life expectancy of a human is usually longer than that of a gorilla.

On the basis of evolution theory, the likeness between humans and monkeys doesn't mean that a human is the same as a monkey. However it does mean that we have a common ancestor with monkeys being around for millions of years, but now, the human is a totally different species.

The deviance of man from his natural diet is obvious in all parts of the world and in all traditions, as we see that even nomads in Africa cook their foods, use salt and most of them are very superstitious as much as they victimize their child in certain ceremonies. So it is not reliable to say that eating insects in some tribes and some countries is a natural human instinct. And on the other hand, we see that these actions are forbidden in some religions and traditions.

Scientific research has so far not found any benefits of eating insects for humans. It is doubtful that any will be found as insects, like raw meat, are full of parasites, so they can be very dangerous for humans.

In tropical countries like Thailand, there are very different delicious tropical fruits. I tasted all Asian tropical fruits when I was in Malaysia. They are very delicious and rich in nutrients. Also the tropical weather is always rainy, and tropical countries have very fertilized soil, which means that they don't have problems such as lack of water or food. But I really don't know the reason why some tribes in Thailand and neighboring countries eat insects or even monkeys' brains, which still continues today. I cannot understand why humans would do such a thing when he has access to the best kinds of fruits and live in the best and most pleasurable climate. Maybe this is not caused by a reaction to a lack of food, but that they are influenced by a behavior deviation or some superstitious ceremonies which are usually caused by fake religious beliefs.

The human body's dietary needs, in order to remain healthy, are covered by natural raw veganism; consuming fruits and vegetables, absorbing sunlight, and drinking clean water.

Now there are some people in the world who have been 100% raw vegan for more than 30 or 40 years and they don't have any deficiency problem, while the average age gorillas and monkeys live to is about 30 to 50 years. So there is no reason for humans to tease themselves by eating unsavory foods.

Some people think that if a person wants to be a vegetarian, he should eat all day long like a gorilla or other herbivores such as a cow. But this is not necessary because firstly, humans are not ruminators and only have one stomach, not two.

And secondly humans have access to a wide range of foods which all differ in calorie content. For example, vegetables are a source of minerals while they are low in calories, while fruit, the main source of energy for humans, is high in calories and other natural foods like nuts contain fat and are full of calories.

So, our natural food is very different from grasses which aren't digestible as they are hard and full of fiber (cellulose), so the ruminators have a two-part stomach to extract nutrients from these hard grasses through the chemical actions of useful bacteria in their abdomen. However they use only some part of nutrients in grass and repulse most of it.

In contrast fruits are very simple to digest for humans, so are very time-saving for us to eat and digest.

Also we should never forget that cooking is a very time consuming process, and this is the true reason why nowadays most people go to restaurants or fast food stores, because as the modern lifestyle made people very busy, they cannot continue their life and their business if they want to also spend time cooking at home. Fortunately, we do not have such a problem with eating fruit. Raw veganism can be a really time-saving diet, as it was for me.

In the book Raw Secrets by Frederic Patenaude he made a reasonable comparison between primates and humans, with noteworthy information that I quote here:

"Let's take a closer look at the diet of the primates.

Gorillas — Mountain gorillas primarily eat green vegetation (95%), partly because they don't find much else in their natural surroundings. They eat rare fruits in season.

According to Dr. George Schaller, a very serious researcher and primatologist in this field, and Dian Fossey, another great primatologist, they do not eat any animal products. In experiments conducted at the San Diego Zoo, gorillas were given the choice between fruit or greens. The results were very interesting. The gorillas in the experiment ended up eating only fruit for the duration of the three months of the experiment.

Chimpanzees — Chimpanzees eat mostly fruits, some green leaves, nuts and sometimes meat. Animal products represent less than about 5% of their diet.

Orangutans — Orangutans eat mostly fruits, some greens, and some nuts. When fruit is rare or not available, they eat more green leaves and some insects. Animal products represent a small portion of their diet. These animals enjoy a wide variety of sweet, delicious fruits, such as rambutan, wild fig and cempedak. They are especially fond of durian.

Bonobos — The bonobos are the closest animals to human beings. They are amazingly similar to us in many ways. Bonobos are now recognized as a separate animal from the chimpanzee. Whereas chimpanzees can be of an aggressive nature, bonobos are calmer and resolve conflicts differently (namely by having sex!). Their diet is also close to our ideal diet: bonobos eat mostly fruits with a certain type of plant similar to sugar cane, as well as various greens, young shoots and buds. They apparently do not eat any nuts. They eat some insects, perhaps small fish and small animals, but they are not seen hunting like chimpanzees. Animal products represent less than 1% of their diet.

It has been difficult to get an idea of what the ideal food for humans is, based on the diets of primates, partly because these eating patterns vary greatly from one type of primate to another and even from tribe to tribe. However, we do know that they all eat a fruit-based diet, except for the gorilla, which apparently would like to differ. They all eat greens in significant quantities. The animal products in their diets are in very small quantities.

Obviously we have similarities with them, so our natural diet should have similarities, but we are not exactly like them, so our diet cannot be exactly like theirs. Note that when chimpanzees eat meat, they can hunt down the animal with their bare hands and eat it freshly killed. Which one of my readers could do the same?"

The potential of the human body

The human body has enough fat and sugar stores to run 1,200 kilometers. And as an example, Dean Karnazes[16], ultra marathon runner, ran 350 miles (560 km) in 80 hours and 44 minutes without sleep in 2005. He also holds the record for running 200+ miles nonstop.

According to an article in Discover Magazine, humans can outrun nearly every other animal on the planet over long distances[17].

Such examples show the real endurance of humans but unfortunately we damage ourselves by eating the wrong foods and not getting enough exercise.

There was evidence and documented research that humans can remain alive without food for more than 20, 40 or even 70 days[18]. (This is not recommended as it can be very dangerous).

How much food do we need?

In the experiences of most raw vegans, consuming 1.5 to 2 kilograms of sweet fruits per day (on average) is enough for every person with an average-sized body who has an average physical activity level. We need a small amount of nuts and seeds and also a healthy amount of vegetables in our diet. It is very economical because in this state each raw vegan will consume almost 700 kilograms of foods each year, and if he/she fasts sometimes or reduces the volume of food for health reasons, the total volume of foods consumed will be decreased even more. According to research by nutrition experts, each person on average eats about 1,000 kilograms of food every year.[19] So we see on the basis of statistics that raw vegans eat less than cooked food eaters and the reason is clear; because they don't waste their food and set fire to the nutrients, so they don't have to eat more to compensate for deficiencies.

Of course in the first few days of starting a raw vegan diet, you will feel a strong hunger and need more food in the beginning because the body is starting to cleanse itself and cells are starting to recover, which is natural and temporary. Also you will experience a severe fake hunger feeling which will disappear after continuing raw veganism. False hunger is the body's attempt to eliminate toxins and regenerate in the region of the stomach and alimentary canal. A necessary process since we are usually overloading it by eating too much, too frequently or unnatural foods[20].

We experience false hunger when we desire food even though our body has no need for it. False hunger is often brought on by a stimulated appetite. Our appetite can be stimulated by condiments, spices, salt, sugar and other flavoring agents that are often added to our foods. These additives provide virtually no nutrition whatsoever. When we are attracted to food merely because of a stimulated appetite, we are not experiencing true hunger. We are only being drawn to eat for recreational purposes, not for any physiological need.[21]

Nature's evolution system: herbivores and carnivores

There are different theories about the food chain and the reason why each animal likes and chooses some foods or which phenomenon causes them to be carnivores. Maybe we could not determine or prove which opinion is absolutely true because evolution on earth took millions and millions of years, hundreds of times longer than humans have existed on earth. So it is necessary to do more research and study to understand the natural system completely.

In the book Raw-Eating by Ter-Hovanessian, he writes about an amazing experiment and theory on carnivorous animals which is very interesting. He says:

"There are very different kinds of herbs and all animals on earth are herbivores. Natural food for all animals is herbal foods, but from old ages, in winters, when natural foods became rare, some animals hibernated, some of them migrated to other places, some stocked foods and some animals ate other animals.

However carnivores eat living meats with living cells, but even this food isn't perfect because it has lost some of its primary nutritive value, and this is the real reason that carnivores sometimes eat herbs while naive people think that carnivores do this action only when they are sick.

All kinds of meats are toxic foods and so, the meat of a carnivore can't be a suitable food for another animal because it is very toxic as much as the effects of its poisons appears immediately, and this is the reason why humans don't dare to eat the meats of carnivores like dogs, cats, lions and tigers.

We can easily ascertain that meat eating isn't natural. My daughter Anahid has a six-year-old beautiful dog which we fed raw vegan foods from birth. Its diet consisted of date palm, grains, raisins and different salads and fruits. All of these foods are raw because it's impossible to find even one gram of dead food in our home! This dog even ate onion and radish with enthusiasm! When we go out of the city with this dog, it grazes on grasslands like a lamb. This dog is very healthy, very merry and energetic in comparison with other dogs.

If we want to introduce the babies of lions, tigers and wolves to vegetarianism, they will leave their voracity after several generations and become manageable. But we can't force sheep and cows to eat meats."

When I read the above text for the first time, it was very hard for me to accept that a dog could become an herbivore and also be energetic without eating meat. But it is a true story and I asked some people who were close friends with Hovanessain during this time and they said that his dog was really very energetic and different from other dogs.

This is not just the case with dogs but also sometimes other carnivorous animals. In the case of pandas, scientists had carried out research to determine why Pandas were vegetarian and how they had adjusted to a vegetarian diet, while they were built like omnivores with short intestines. They found that: "pandas' digestive tracts do in fact contain bacteria similar to those in the intestines of herbivores," and that: "Even with help from gut bugs, pandas don't derive much nutrition from bamboo—a panda digests just 17 percent of the 20 to 30 pounds (9 to 14 kilograms) of dry food it eats each day. This explains why pandas also evolved a sluggish, energy-conserving lifestyle." [22]

However, some researchers believe that carnivores are completely adjusted to eating meat and they have a very important role in nature because they control the population of animals which in turn increases the efficiency of natural sources by removing weak and damaged animals. They also help to balance the ecosystem because it controls the populations of herbivores.[23]

As we see in nature and wildlife, carnivores should eat flesh certainly and if they couldn't access meat, they would die from starvation. If it was possible for them to survive with herbs, they would eat herbs in emergency situations, but they don't.

Of course there may be some exceptions which we so far cannot explain such as the "world's first vegetarian shark". This is a shark which became vegetarian after a wound in her mouth caused by a fishing hook.[24]

But our purpose is not to change all carnivores on earth to herbivores. Because carnivores are also useful for the environment as they help to line breed and also help to keep the balance between the populations of different kinds of creatures. However, there is some evidence to suggest that even carnivores were maybe herbivores originally, as it seems that some carnivores changed to herbivores during millions years of evolution[25].

We don't know how animals see the world, so we should respect their lives and instead, improve ourselves and make peace. Our mental and philosophical reasoning steers us to avoid any kind of violence so we have to follow this inner guide. If we do that, we do not need to decide for animals.

Carnivores can be divided into two groups: the group which chases its prey and kills it (like lions and tigers), and another group which only eat dead corpses, like vultures. They are very useful for the environment because the decaying corpses become home to dangerous microbes which can risk the lives of all creatures, but these corpse eating animals eat them, thus helping to clean the environment. They don't damage themselves because their stomach acidity and other parts of their body kill fatal microbes.

Or when cats eat mice, it is very beneficial for us, because mice are harmful for human food supplies, and even with all the methods of preventing it, there are millions of tons of human food eaten by mice every year. Just imagine if mice didn't have any predators... they would eat everything.

Perhaps some changes will occur in the future as evolution continues. For example carnivores act as population controllers of other animals, but if creatures can control their population in other ways, the role of carnivores could be changed in the future.

Some people believe that dogs are omnivores, not carnivores, so they can become completely vegan. However, it is a point of debate[26]. And of course keeping pets in houses and separating them from nature has many consequences but if anyone wants to make his/her dog vegan, it is better to note new recommendations[27]. These include the advice that some foods can be harmful for dogs like onions and raisins (despite what Hovanessian experienced!).

Some advantages of a vegan diet

I would like to talk about some of the advantages of a vegan diet[28]:

Avoid antibiotics: antibiotics are almost always given to (non-organic) feed animals, which can lead to bacterial resistance in humans. Many of the antibiotics used to treat human infections are also used to feed animals. This means by consuming this, we are causing ourselves to be less resistant to antibiotics.

Appropriate puberty: since 1950, girls are hitting puberty on average 4-7 years earlier and boys' sperm counts have decreased by 25-50% due to the hormones present in non-organic meat and dairy products.

Reduced risk of Alzheimer's: meat eaters have double the rate of Alzheimer's disease as vegans.

Reduce your risk of cancer: vegans have a 40% reduced chance of developing cancer than the general population which is thought to be because they have a higher intake of vitamins A, C & E.

Eliminate bad cholesterol: eliminate any food that comes from an animal and you will eliminate all of the 'bad' dietary cholesterol from your diet (heart disease is the leading cause of death in America today).

As early as 1961, The AMA journal stated that 90+% of heart disease can be prevented with a vegetarian diet.

There is a strong link between colon cancer and meat-eating because the toxins in meat are not expelled as quickly they would be in carnivores.

Dioxin, one of the deadliest toxins, is concentrated in meat at levels 22 times above what is considered safe. According to the Environmental Protection Agency (EPA), more than 95% of all dioxin exposure comes from meat, dairy, and eggs. None are found in vegan foods (the other 5% is environmental).

Also Mad Cow Disease is really "The Man's Greed Disease". Cows were fed the remains of other animals, which was put in their feed to save money. Being herbivorous, cows have 4 stomachs, and animal matter rotted in their system and caused the disease.

What about protein? How do the rhino, the elephant and the bull survive? Inadequacy of protein in a vegetarian diet is a complete myth propagated by people with vested interests. In fact, over-ingestion of protein in the Western diet has been detrimental to our health. However grains, beans, sprouts and nuts are all concentrated sources of protein. Lentils contain more protein per ounce than hamburger, pork or steak.

Increase your energy: when following a healthy vegan diet, you will find your energy is much higher.

On the basis of the reasons which show us that humans are vegan by his anatomy, and also by the philosophy and experiences of Khorsand concerning raw eating, it seems there are many facts which are unknown to us that we should try to find. But a different view about nourishment and trying to find the truth isn't limited only to some special people.

Research and views of Arshavir Ter-Hovanessian

Arshavir Ter-Hovanessian is the Armenian-Iranian founder of Raw Eating veganism in Iran and author of the book 'Raw eating, or, A New World free from diseases, vices and poisons.' The first part of the book was published in 1962.

He became familiar with veganism after reading a book about diseases caused by inappropriate nutrition from Bircher Benner, a famous German researcher in the field of nourishment. Reading this book helped Arshavir to reach a different view about the cause of diseases and discover the main cause of all sicknesses. After his two babies died from diseases and he was suffering different diseases himself at the age of 54, he discovered (like Khorsand) that the real cause of all diseases was cooked food which destroys most vital nutrients while producing toxins in the food. He also discovered with eating cooked and baked foods, hunger pangs intensified.

I have translated parts of this book which I think are note worthy.

In the beginning of the book Raw Eating by Arshavir Ter-Hovanessian (ATerHov) we read:

"Dead food means disease and death, while living food means complete health and long life.

Dead eaters don't bake foods in the kitchen, they bake diseases!

Baking perishes all the vital and necessary materials in the food and makes it toxic.

Desire for dead food isn't a true appetite; it's the mendacious appetite that an addict feels for toxic things.

An awful age will end with the end of dead eating.

A blessed age will start with the start of live eating.

No one can reach a natural old age in the dead eating age, all people perish from diseases. In the live eating time, no one will perish by diseases, but also all people will reach old age and how long will a human lifetime be? 200 or 300 years? No one knows, because it hasn't been seen yet.

Those are dangerous madcaps and enemies of humankind who frighten people with unreal danger of a lack of foods. Lack of foods doesn't exist in this world, but the "civilized" people waste eighty percent of natural foods through cooking. If grains were only used in a raw and natural state by everyone, most of it will be surplus. This is a fact."

A message for athletes

In the aforementioned book of A-Ter-Hov, we read:
"Dear athletes!
You have been misinformed. Baked foods and especially "animal proteins" not only don't give you power and merriment, but also it wastes your energy, and instead of sports being good for you, the wearing out of your body is accelerated with these foods and you are forced to leave sports in your youth at the ages of 30-35 years, and after that you are forced to add to the society of lazy dead eaters with a worn out body.

Anyone who is wise, should relinquish dead foods immediately, and rescue his/her body from toxins, reinforce muscles with natural foods and go to the competition field with a fresh power to get unprecedented rewards.

Real live food eaters will increase their physical body and mental power day by day for a long time, longer than what is imagined (100, 120 years or even more).

Live eaters don't linger for a taxi or bus, they walk and reach their destination quicker and this is one solution to reduce traffic. But a dead eating youth lingers for a bus for half an hour instead of walking for ten minutes, shame on them!"

An important lesson

Reading such sentences for the first time makes us surprised because they are the opposite of what we have learnt and heard before.

However we know that several centuries ago, people thought the earth was flat or that the sun moved around the earth. Now we know the truth but for many of us, we have not learnt the most important lesson of history: <u>do not repeat mistakes of the past.</u>

So here we are in 21st century where many people do not want to accept different ideas because they don't want to change their habits and opinions.

Now is the time to understand the reality of the situation, to broaden our horizons and have the ability to see and accept more than our limited knowledge. This is the only way to reach emancipation.

Rethinking our nutrition

Do you think there is no deficiency in our knowledge and humans know all the facts about nutrition?

Different modern diseases are evidence which show that our knowledge is very defective, such limited knowledge is not reliable enough for us.

Like many other people, I thought for several years that what we are told about proteins, vitamins, minerals, etc. is true and my belief was that at least we can trust new sciences because they are perfect and exact, but after reading the book of A. T. Hovannessian, my viewpoint changed and the more research I did, the more I became convinced that human knowledge was even more limited than what I had already thought.

Even raw foodists need to rethink and research more about some theories, like the live food enzyme theory.

Now I would like to share more experiences of Arshavir Ter-Hovanessian. If I write such sentences with my name, I think it's not fair because I found these facts in a book which was published two decades before I was born. So I share this noteworthy information with you while I revere copyright, as my purpose is to share what I know.

Also please note that I don't want to idolize Hovanessian. Nothing and nobody is perfect, but we can still extract very useful information from his books, which are credible even today.

In his book Hovanessian writes about what scientists said about human nourishment from the beginning until the book was published 40 years ago. I don't agree with all of his statements but I think most of them are still interesting. Hovanessian writes:

"Everything said about proteins, vitamins, minerals, etc. until now, is wrong and we have to ignore them.

If we suppose (because no one knows about it exactly) that humans or animals need 10,000 kinds of necessary edible materials, all these materials exist in each kind of edible plants, however we cannot see all vitamins and other vital materials in only one kind of herb, but the body can change the materials in the food and make other necessary materials. This is the reason that we see other mammals like sheep, camels or elephants supply all of their body's needs with only one kind of herb without any problems.

But we should not forget that this is true only for raw vegetables, not cooked and dead foods."

Some of Hovannessian statements have been denied today, but still human knowledge is very limited and it is very obvious.

Is it really possible to supply all the human body's needs with only one kind of herb?

This theory is debatable as there isn't much research on this subject. So I asked nutritionist Dr. Zarin Azar, one of the most recognized researchers on nourishment and also a member of PCRM (Physicians Committee for Responsible Medicine) and she answered:

"Not much is known about this subject because not much research has taken place and also many materials in plants and the human body are still unknown. But it is clear that the human body and nature are intelligent and the body really can change some materials into food and make essential materials. However, this theory that the human body can remain healthy while consuming only one kind of vegetable perhaps may be impossible in this age because of the negative effects of environmental pollutants, climate change, using different chemical fertilizers and herbicides on plants. The human body can get all the essential and vital materials it needs using different plants including fruits, vegetables, nuts and seeds."[29]

But as we see in nature each animal has access to a limited variety of foods, which are its main foods. Sometimes animals eat some kinds of herb (of course in small amounts) which are not their main food, such as medical herbs. For example it's well-known that if a horse gets bitten by a snake, it will search for special kinds of herbs which neutralize snake venom (horses do this innately).

During the three years of being a vegan, I have only heard two cases of a mono-diet, where you eat only one kind of plant for a long time. One of these cases was an Iranian youth who ate only apples for 6 months and he said he felt better and more detoxed. He said he never felt bored during this time and shared his experiences through an Iranian raw food group on Facebook.

The other case was a raw vegan, again from Iran, who tried to live only on watermelons for four years due to financial problems but became very weak and suffered many deficiencies, including anemia and B12 deficiency. But after that, he stopped this mono diet and started to eat all different raw plant foods, and as result his health improved.

Fortunately we have access to different kinds of fruits and vegetables, so it is very easy to be a healthy vegan or a raw vegan. Some medical herbs can be useful for us in particular cases, as animals use these herbs occasionally. (Please note that these herbs can't be used as a replacement for the main food and also using them daily causes negative side effects so it's better not to use them until it is necessary or in an emergency situation).

The dangerous effects of cooked foods on the body

Today we are more familiar with the human body along with its similarities and differences with other animals, but our knowledge is still very limited.

We have explored how dead foods can be harmful for each animal, due to the experiences discussed by Mr. Khorsand covered in previous pages.

Now it is clear that one of the important factors in all human diseases is eating cooked and junk foods.

I would like to refer to another part of the book "Raw-Eating" by Ter-Hovanessian:

"All diseases are the result of involving dead-foods and other unnatural and toxic materials to the body.

Dead food burns like a useless fuel in the body and creates useless cells and causes the person to gain unnecessary extra weight, which some misinformed people count as power. Also, dead foods produce different poisons which become congested in the human body over long periods and cause innumerable diseases.

Diseases are produced from eating dead and toxic foods such as all cooked foods, all animal foods, chemical drugs, all narcotic, soft drinks and alcoholic drinks, tobacco, sugar and so on.

The appetite which anyone feels for dead foods isn't the real relish; it's a mendacious appetite such as an addict would feel for toxic materials. He fills his stomach with dead foods to feel full, while his body groans from the intensity of real hunger!

In the body of every dead food eating person, there are two kinds of cells: the main cells and the useless cells.

Eating natural live (raw) food causes the creation of healthy and specialist cells, while unnatural and dead-foods create weak, sick and hanger-on cells! All human diseases are concentrated in these useless cells. Sometimes the weight of these useless cells reach even 70 kg and this is the exact disease which embraces the person and controls him!

Generally, disease means a lack of main and expert cells in the body plus the addition of useless cells and different toxins in the body.

When the number of the main and expert cells in the kidneys, which clean up the blood, diminishes and kidneys stop working properly, we say that the kidneys are sick.

Or when the main cells in the liver decrease, we say that the liver is sick and this can be said for other organs in the body.

When a patient becomes familiar with this fact and decides to heal his or her self, they cut off using all dead foods, start to eat natural and healthy foods, thus killing the useless cells in his or her body and various stored poisons start dissolving from the first day he starts live eating. The real cells become stronger and increase day by day and as a result, glands and organs in the body return to their natural duties. He or she reaches better health in a miraculous manner within a short period of time.

I ask you which "medicine" can kill useless cells, empty the body from poisons or nourish the hungry and the real cells? When I walk in front of drug stores and see how these people waste their money buying such drugs which harm their body more, I want to scream and warn them about the perils of their actions. These poisons should be collected from pharmacies and shown in museums for future generations to see how we lived in the 20th century and the effect on our health as a result of such pernicious poisons!

Foods for humans should be made from live cells. There is no nutritional value in dead foods.

Carnivores use herbal materials indirectly from raw meats of herbivores, no heating required, but the majority of us cannot eat animals raw, as we can eat herbs, therefore humans cannot be natural meat eaters."

Ter-Hovanessian goes on to explain why eating meat is harmful, even if it is raw.

"Perhaps you ask: "How can Eskimos eat raw meats and they are almost healthy?"

The answer to this question is that it seems Eskimos fell into the habit of eating raw meats (fish) as a result of their glacial environment and lack of plant foods. Due to the fact they eat meats in a raw state containing whole nutrients, enzymes and other vital materials, they don't have many modern diseases but still they aren't immune from poisons in meats so as a result, Eskimos have short statures and generally shorter life spans than the average human. Eating raw meat can also increase the risk of getting parasites.

What is worth noting is the natural meats which Eskimos eat isn't comparable with junk foods, cold cuts or frankfurters which are full of hormones and other chemical poisons! These are pure poisons!

You can't expect to eat these (junk) foods and expect to remain healthy! But when we become sick we often think it is nature at odds with our body.

Is this nature's fault when we destroy our foods and turn them into dangerous foods and eat them?! If we don't treat nature kindly how can we expect nature to be kind to us?!"

I would like to include more quotes from the book "Raw-eating" which supports this view that dead foods create useless cells. He also talks about the cause of diseases and how we make them disappear. He writes:

"Dead foods, especially animal foods, produce different toxins which permeate to all parts of the body and these toxins congregate in the body after several years and cause diseases like gout, arteriosclerosis, hypertension, kidney stones and so on. The number of main cells in organs and glands decrease because of a lack of natural healthy food, so organs cannot do their duty well.

Now let us look at the causes of heart disease which is the most common cause of death in humans.

We can liken blood flow to a city's water system. If anyone off-loads a large amount of trash in the water system, the trash will block part of the pipeline and will cut off the water flow. Similarly, when people add toxins to their blood every day during breakfast, lunch and dinner, these poisons settle on the blood vessels day by day gradually restricting these vessels and eventually can cut off the blood flow completely with dire consequences.

Small-minded people class this as a sudden death. If that person could see the continual dumping of waste into their own system that person wouldn't refer to such an event as "sudden".

When I see how these incognizant people put toxins into their body by eating beef, fish, eggs and cheese, I'm appalled that at any moment their blood flow may stop, and this unlucky event could happen.

Heart failure has another cause too. As I said earlier, most cells in the bodies of dead food eaters produced from eating dead foods aren't reactionary so they can't fulfill their duty well. Your heart increases blood pressure because of the vessels' constriction to it and can supply blood to the endmost points of the body. Weak partitions of vessels especially vessels in the brain, can't handle this high blood pressure so they crack.

Doctors tend to use chemical drugs instead of advising not to eat certain foods. The drugs doctors use dilute blood with chemical materials, activating vessels with different poisons and dilate them for only a few days, adding more toxins to the already weak heart and forcing it to collect its last powers and work a little faster. After using some plates of "strengthening" dead foods like barbecue, everything returns to its previous status, but with the difference that the weak heart weakens even more, some new poisons add to previous poisons in the body and some new money is added to the income of doctors and pharmacists!

For example, when treating hypertension, doctors sometimes prescribe a toxin which dilates vessels in an artificial manner. So after a while, the heart will become tired because it's working in excess and it can become bigger, and although it continues to function fully, it weakens as your blood pressure decreases to lower than its normal state. To treat this issue drugs such as "Vasodilatatores" and "Vasoconstrictors" are used which straitens the vessels and puts more force on the heart. These toxins produce other poisons to activate the tired organs which work slowly and want to rest a little, and force them to work faster.

What is important to note is that Nature doesn't put pressure on organs in the human body. For example, removing tonsils is a common operation, but we should know that nature put tonsils in the human body to combat harmful micro-organisms. When tonsils start their battle with harmful micro-organisms, the doctor, who sees only the outward result of this, removes the tonsils which are one of the most important defensive castles of the body, instead of helping them and destroying the main enemy.

Cooked and dead foods can contribute to thousands of human disorders. These dead foods, in one case can affect protein metabolism in a manner which makes the person very skinny or in other cases could adds several kilos of useless fat to the body.

Scientists have published countless books and held countless conferences on the uses of different artificial hormones and drugs, but they don't want to consider one simple thing; that if we bring in natural food into the body, the body will work in its natural state. Anyone who doesn't understand the meaning of the word natural doesn't understand anything at all!

Now cancer is the most astounding subject. It's ascertainable for scientists that cancer is the baby of dead foods, but they don't want to tell people this truth, perhaps they don't want to deprive people of the "enjoyment" of these "delicious" and "life-giving" foods when they are life-giving for cancerous cells.

Of course some doctors do recommend the natural way to treat cancer and they have got nice results, but unfortunately most doctors don't want to inform everyone of this fact, why? Because cancer treatment drugs, as an industry, is worth billions of dollars.

Because of a lack of natural and healthy foods, the main body cells can't prevent the growth of cancerous and useless cells, but when we stop using dead foods thoroughly, all useless cells, whether cancerous cells or extra fat cells, starve and will disappear.

Why do "doctors" and "scientists" not see this very easy truth? Many cannot see how nature creates a great tree from a very small seed or creates big animals like camels and elephants from microscopic ingredients.

They destroy all conclusions which nature produced over millions of years in their labs and instead, produce different kinds of mortal poisons and splurge them!

I should like to reiterate all diseases are due to the consumption of dead foods and chemical materials which threaten the human health in these three ways:

Aggregation of toxic materials which are introduced to the human body through dead-foods.

The lack of healthy cells in the body, which are caused by a lack of natural foods in the body.

Aggregation of extra and useless cells which are produced from dead-foods.

Toxic materials pervade in all parts of the body and cause damage. The number of active cells in organs decreases because of the shortage of natural healthy food and as extra useless cells disturb their correct function.

The human body is made up of billions of cells. Each cell is a great factory with many advanced and arranged organs that manage our bodies. For example, nerve cells send orders from the mind to our organs as fast as electricity, or muscle cells, which have a resilient ability, can move and raise heavy bulks. Cells in our glands produce different hormones, enzymes and other fluids. Heart cells have a special recessive ability which moves the heart in a continual manner. Kidney cells purify blood with their special organs and repulse harmful materials of the blood via urine. Lung cells get oxygen from the air and eject carbon dioxide and dirty air out of body. As such, each cell in each organ has a special duty that if these duties are executed properly according to natural laws, humans can live without any diseases during a long lifetime which God (the creator) determines. And humankind should have a lifetime which is much longer than other creatures because he is the most equipped and the most advanced creature on Earth, but unfortunately most of us reach the ages of 70 or 80 and think we are old therefore sudden death isn't unnatural.

Most of the poisons which accumulate in the human body and cause diseases are produced from animal foods. Also when we put dead animals on a fire, all materials which are essential for the inner structures of expert cells are destroyed and only calories remain, like protein, starch, fats and sugar, which are spoilt by cooking too.

Now let's see what these spoilt foods do to the human body:

Calories produced from dead-foods are useless, like an extra fuel which the body doesn't need and tries to eject. When we eat such foods we feel very hot which triggers an abnormal thirst which we try to pacify with a cold drink. The extra water isn't needed by the body so it prompts the heart to work faster and forward this water to the kidneys and the surface of the skin to eject it by urine and perspiration causing him or her to sweat more."

Hovanessian experiences

Arshavir Ter-Hovannessian wrote about his own health and how it was affected by eating dead foods saying:

"I was involved in these bad situations for 53 years. Each year, I had a cold two or three times and each time, for three or four days. I had been sweating so much that my underpants streamed with perspiration in only 10-12 minutes. After changing my underpants four or five times, I had been tired and wore a bath towel before I would go to bed.

I had chronic bronchitis for 25 years, which was very hard and I had a feeling like there was a hole in my chest which cold air always enters my body from.

I wore thick jackets and thick Ascots but they were useless; cold air was finding a way to enter my chest.

Sixteen years ago I became wise and started eating live foods. I slept in the fresh air whether in summer or winter, and always cold air bops with my body but I didn't get sick because of this cold air.

Now I don't wear pajamas when I go to sleep. In winter, I wear underclothing, but in summer, I don't even wear this undershirt and I sleep under a bed sheet to let my skin breathe freely. I wet my body with a glass of water or shower before bed in the very hot nights of summer, so I feel an enjoyable coolness which enables me to sleep deeply immediately.

As we said, when we kill live foods with fire, those primary materials which are vital for the formation of cells and their organs, are destroyed and only useless calories and heavy materials remain. We've explored the effects of extra calories, now we will look at the effects of such heavy materials on the body.

Protein from foods such as meats, (baked) rice and bread can only produce a parapet of cells. These cells are similar to main cells apparently, but they haven't any special organs so the only thing they can do is eat and digest foods and reproduce. Not one of the main cells in the body is jobless; each of them has a special duty and they do their duties in the skin, bones, organs and glands. (Perhaps I'm insane and I don't understand anything, now you tell me what the benefit is of these extra cells from eating meats and fats which are dangling off the bodies of dead food eaters?!)

I would now like to explore the term 'sickness'. When someone feels an ache in his or her legs, head or heart, or has a fever, we say that this person got sick, while in fact, this is not true. The root of the sickness is as a result of three factors; the aggregation of poisons in the body, a production of extra cells and a lack of expert cells, so all dead food eaters without any exception are sick, from a one-day-old baby (which was nourished in the womb of its mother with dead foods) to men and women more than 100 years old, all of them are sick.

Now perhaps you ask me: "if that's not sickness which forces someone to stay in bed for months and even years, then what is it?" and my answer is as follows:

Those discomforts which dead food eaters sometimes feel aren't real sicknesses but instead they are the symbols of resistance of the body against dead foods.

When someone eats dead foods regularly, their bodies become tired and sometimes struggle to remove harmful materials from the body, so the body often empties the stomach by being sick, cleans the bowel by diarrhea and, and can also reduce the appetite for four to five days to let the digestive system have a short rest. So, vomit and diarrhea are not symptoms of a sickness; in fact, these are symptoms of treatment! Sometimes nature causes such reactions to try and drive out some parts of the disease from the body.

Dogmatic dead food eaters don't understand this and instead of letting nature take its course, instead of letting their digestive system have a rest, which worked for decades three to four times more than it should, instead of removing dead and poisonous foods from their food program and empowering their body with natural foods, they try to prevent the remedial struggle of nature with different kinds of poisonous medicines and "scientific" tools, and with chicken soup or cow's milk, empowering the sick body instead of our natural state!

This struggle can be seen in all kinds of illnesses. Fever and feeling pain are signs of a struggle of the main body against different poisons and microbes.

Dead food eating biologists invented thousands of different scientific names for the desolations caused by eating dead foods. Now let's look at how these desolations pervade the body.

Like water that flows down a mountain and ends up in any free hole it finds in its way when a person produces toxic foods in the kitchen and brings them into the body, these materials go everywhere they find a free cavity or weak point. Sometimes these poisons find a weak organ along the way and begin to destroy it. In some cases this can affect a person at a young age. In other cases, these desolations pervade all organs of the body and the person gets lucky and continues to live into their 80s or 90s. In the view of dead food eaters, this is a long life!

It's difficult to say why some people die from these conditions earlier or later because it depends on the use of dead and live foods, the health of their organs, their job situation, personal life or genetics.

Dead food eaters consider these diseases as part of civilization without a clear understanding of what is the true cause.

Those things that dead eaters count as civilization such as companies that produce fast foods, cigarettes, liquors, chemical medicines, stoves and many other tools that half-crazy people invented to turn natural foods into poisonous materials and eradicate generations of humans, not only are these not symbols of civilization, but also this is the biggest barbarism in today's world.

If we look back 200, 300 years, cancer and heart disease were considered maladies of old age, but now babies are born with cancer and people in their 20s die from heart attacks.

Think about that! No number of operations, wealth and power can prevent these misfortunes except changing a plate of dead food to a plate of live food, which is determined by the creator of all creations.

Look at these deluxe hospitals equipped with complex scientific devices. I think that all these useless "scientific" actions put together haven't got the power of one plate of live food.

Everyone who wants to learn something in particular will read and repeat it several times to remember it. As live eating and the philosophy of nourishment and health is the most important lesson in this world, it's necessary to remember and repeat it every time and everywhere.

When a factory is built its engineer has to determine exactly the materials necessary and what is going to keep it a secure and safe. Now let us turn to the human body, the greatest factory in this world, and who created it or its engineer? If biologists have created our brains, hearts and lungs, so we are compelled to follow their directions, and if our bodies have another engineer, we should know him and follow his directions.

Everyone in this world who worships God and imagines him in their mind believes that the main engineer of our bodies is God. Can we speak with God? Of course yes! God isn't sitting in a special place; he is everywhere, in the sky, on Earth, in our hearts, in our brain, in a seed of wheat, in flowers, in leaves, in the eyes of cows, sheep, and hens. So, God speaks with us through nature every minute of the day. Even those people who don't know God and do not believe in him, know nature and so believe in God in other forms, because God shows himself in all places of nature and we should accept that "God", "the Creator" and "nature" have the same meaning. Nature has special rules that are written on all things in this world and if biologists really want to do something useful, they should find and read these rules carefully and help people to find the true way.

In this part of the book I talked about the three factors; extra cells, poisonous materials and lack of the main cells being the main cause of all diseases and when we stop eating dead foods, extra cells and poisons exit the body and the main cells become stronger and start their natural duties. But while eradicating these poisons and extra cells the body reacts in a way which many health experts do not recognize and instead diagnose it incorrectly. This is the root of all errors in medical sciences, and in the next part of this book I will explain such reactions. (Remedial reactions in the next page).

Remedial Reactions

We have said that sickness is the symptom of the body's struggle against alien and poisonous materials which enter the body.

When many more poisons are produced from dead foods, if the body can't save it or expel it, it remains in the blood stream and the person may experience a headache, stomach ache or other pains. If that person were to then change their diet or experience changes such as hot sun, hot wind etc part of their stored poisons become solved and the person feels the pain. Certain people may refer to these pains as "sickness", when actually these are the symptoms of the main malady. This pain is from the main body which screams and requests help from us, but narrow-minded doctors stifle this inner voice with several chemical and paregoric medicines instead of helping the body. They only add new poisons to existing poisons!

Now I request from you to read this section carefully and remember it well and don't have any doubt about it.

When a person stops using dead foods and uses natural foods, these foods show their sanative effects immediately. Natural foods help drive out non-digested and dead foods which are wandering in the intestines and also in the blood, so the person (maybe) feels some pain in his/her intestine such as gas, diarrhea and so on. If he doesn't know the facts, he thinks the natural foods have harmed him! This is very funny! It shouldn't be called natural if it sickens the body. Many people don't read this subject carefully and tell me: "We tried raw eating, but we saw that natural foods aren't suitable for our bodies so we gave up."

The poisons which haven't yet become solid and are fluid, start to leave the body after weeks and months, but those ones which entered the body a decade ago or earlier will be firm like stones so it takes several years to soften and change into a fluid state before leaving the body. Most of the severe pains which dead food eaters feel in some parts of their bodies are because of these materials. The poisons can't pass from the cells to the blood stream to eventually be driven out which causes severe pains.

These reactions against alien materials (which people refer to as "sickness") are seen in both the dead food eating period and if a person switches to live food eating. This is because in dead food eating, poisons are put into the body so whatever cannot be driven out is stored in different parts of the body. But in live food eating no more poisons enter the body and it is just stored poisons from previous dead food eating which are being driven out slowly. Therefore, in the case of dead food eating, the body is becoming weaker and the sickness is becoming worse, but in the condition of live food eating, parts of the main malady are driven out after each attack and the person becomes healthier and stronger.

I know many people who say: "my stomach is weak; I can't eat any fruit because if I eat a little fruit or vegetables, I become sick." He doesn't know that not only do fruits not sicken him, but also that they start remedial reactions immediately which clean the intestines and rescue him or her from illness. This person is always sick, he is sick because he has not eaten fruits. He always has indigestion without fruits and vegetables. His body is always struggling and he may lose his appetite to allow his body to empty his stomach of poisons, but the person doesn't realize what is happening and continues to eat as before! If this person goes to a doctor, and say that fruits harm me, what should I do? The response is often: "If you believe that harms you, don't eat it." I doubt any of them would say: "Just try and eat it for ten days then see the result." Of course they never say this because they fear that fruit may be killing the person, but they never consider that meat and dead foods may be the cause of death.

Now if I say this "very small" mistake caused all global wars and all modern murders, narrow-minded people will laugh at me, such as four hundred and fifty years ago when they were laughing at Nicolaus Copernicus because he said that the Earth was moving. There are also some people who say: "How is fruit not harmful when I see it does me harm because I get diarrhea?!"

But I say and repeat that not only is there a relation but also it is the only reason for all wars. People kill each other to gain a bigger piece of toxic and dead foods. Go to political feasts and see how much money is spent on collecting toxic materials and putting them on smorgasbords instead of the real foods, or go to Asian lands and observe how they filter a million tons of worthy and compressed foods like rice and kill them (by baking) and turn them into scum and put it in front of millions of hungry people instead of real foods.

If this person, who is weak, always has indigestion and suffers health-wise, decides to eat fruits, which he dislikes, but tolerates its remedial reactions for some days, it will rescue him from diseases. For a quick example of how it works, I would like to relay my experience.

I don't think anyone ate meats as much as I did. I only considered I had eaten if my meal was meat. Most of the food I ate was chicken fried drumsticks, fish, barbecued meats and eggs. I didn't even count cheese, milk, yoghurt and butter as foods as I only believed in meats. I was laughing at people who didn't consume meat, alcohol and cigarettes, I thought they were insane!

I didn't abhor eating fruits but those didn't matter for me. When I was filling my belly with meats and fatty foods and I wanted to leave the house, my mother was always asking me: "will you eat some fruit before you go?!" I was always forgetting fruits.

Storing poisons in my body started from childhood, but I was one of the "lucky" people who had poisons in all parts of my body, meaning I had collected tens of different types of diseases.

I suffered all different childhood diseases; rheumatic problems, headaches, insomnia, constipation, diarrhea, several colds, angina, two hard types of typhus, asphyxia, hard hemorrhoid, gout, persistent bronchitis, stomach acidification, atherosclerosis, hypertension, irregular heartbeat and finally hard edema of foots, asthma, prostate disease and countless other maladies which caused me to become near death at age 53 . I was becoming tired after I walked a little distance; I had thought that I had become old. If after my two innocent children died I didn't become wise, I would have died long ago but now I have been reborn and now I understand what real life is.

When I left dead-food eating, I didn't see the remedial reactions in the first few days, perhaps because some poisons had become solid in my body and it took time to leave my body. In the first few days I had a lot of gas and an ache in my intestines which I never minded. But instead, my headaches, insomnia and stomach acidification had almost disappeared after the first few days.

I started walking every day and after a while, I had increased my walking to five or six kilometers a day. I was intentionally walking fast to help eradicate poisons. I felt like my body was overrun with poisons, I had vertigo, I heard loud noises in my ears and I wanted to blast them!

Uric acid is the most dangerous poison which sabotages the human body. When this poison collects in the body's joints and especially in the big toe and prevents them from moving, it becomes gout. The pressure I put on my feet when I was walking caused the uric acid responsible for my gout to disappear. This was very interesting for me, in the age of dead food eating when I was collecting toxins and I felt pain, it felt like somebody was hammering on my big toe but when I switched to live food eating when the poison had left my body I no longer felt the pain.

This is only the beginning of my journey. My body was full of poison which needed to be removed. I have no doubt that some of this poison had left my body without any special suffering, but nevertheless, in the first years of live food eating once or twice each year I would get sick for a few days due to the fact the poisons had moved from my organs to my blood before leaving my body. This process made me feel weak and tired with little appetite and my urine was discolored. I often experienced a fever during these times but I never minded these discomforts and I continued with my life and work, because I had faith in nature and I knew that these reactions had to happen for nature to be able to rescue me. After each reaction and period of sickness I felt ten years younger and so much healthier.

I wasn't very fat (65 kilograms and 165 centimeters) but I lost 12 kilos. All of my friends and acquaintances thought I was insane that unlike them I deprived myself of animal protein and "strengthening", "complete" and "bracing" foods. Unfortunately some of those "fat" and "strong" people, who pitied me more than others, aren't alive today to see the result. My weight has stopped dipping after the last reaction (at least I think so) and I've gained three or four kilos.

Before live food eating, my feet had edema because of my heart disease, a soft and dangerous edema which when I did stick my finger in it, its mark remained for some minutes. In the first years of live food eating, this edema decreased, but it didn't disappear. Two or three years later it suddenly intensified for several months. It is important to note that in most cases, poisons exit the way it first entered. If it started with a headache, it will exit with headache and so on. Of course this is not a rule. One day in AbAli mountains (in north of Tehran province) I was walking under the hot sun, and suddenly I felt vertigo. I got home with difficulty. Edema appeared on my foot, my urine was discolored and the vertigo continued for a while. I was lying on the floor and when I tried to lift my head everything went black, I was close to fainting. When these reactions passed, I felt like I was twenty years younger and my edema decreased slightly. Finally it appeared some years ago for the last time and after that, it disappeared completely.

The most interesting thing was the reactions which appeared in my legs two years ago and then again last year. Three years ago, after almost thirteen years of live food eating, pain similar to rheumatism started in my legs, under the knees, which wasn't too severe but it prevented me from sleeping comfortably at night. This pain continued for seven to eight months until finally one day, when I was kneeling down working in the garden, I stood up and felt a very hard pain so severe that couldn't move from my place. After that, this pain pervaded in all parts of my body and it took seven to eight months to decrease from its intensity slowly and finally disappeared.

Of course I had faith that all of these reactions were from nature which was emptying my body from poisons and maladies, but my amazement was in just how much poisons had been collected during those thirteen years. I thought about this subject very much until finally I remembered that at the age of eighteen, my right leg especially near the knee had got rheumatism which stayed with me for two years. Now I understand that the poisons which entered my body first took more time to leave my body.

The rheumatism meant I couldn't move my right leg very well, it felt like there was something under my knee that was preventing me from squatting. This was the uric acid which had been stuck there for more than fifty years. After I changed my diet and the poisons had exited my body I was able to move my right leg freely.

Reactions such as these are also observed in dead food eaters. The aching of body joints are the poisons which are stored between the joints (more in the waistline and spine) and sometimes they break into an abnormal movement and produce such a hard pain that the person can't move anymore. Removing this pain can be done in two completely opposite manners. One way is to clean the body from uric acid to let the blood eradicate the poisons. Another way is eating fish, meat and eggs and increasing the level of uric acid in the blood so the decomposed poisons can't solve in it and it returns to its early point. It depends on the mind of the doctor or the person to decide the path they take. The medical test to calculate the level of uric acid in the blood or urine isn't useful because no one can distinguish whether this uric acid has recently entered the body or it was already stored in the body. And more importantly, no one can calculate the amount of uric acid which is stored in the organs of dead food eaters. Some readers think that I have suffered from these reactions frequently.

The reactions which can be considered as painful, took place five to six times in total which were no longer than four or five days each time. This (in total) twenty five days of suffering is very little compared to angina or other diseases which I suffered while I was eating dead food.

These reactions don't follow a special rule. They depend on the volume of stored poisons and their locations. Maybe these remedial reactions in some people were more severe than a usual sickness, because the poisons which are gradually collected over several years are now suddenly solved. In 20-25 year-olds who haven't collect many poisons and extra cells, the reactions may happen without any obvious symptoms, but in older people, it is hard and vigorous.

Unfortunately some people don't read this subject matter carefully and after a few days following their switch to live eating, when the reactions start, they think that the natural foods harmed them! So they get scared and go to the doctor. Narrow-minded doctors count those signs of treatment as harmful signs and return the "sick" to dead-eating. Sometimes this silliness is dangerous as some doctors strongly forbid most patients from eating live fruits and vegetables. In doing so they deprive people of natural food with drastic consequences.

Especially those people who are afraid of fruits who think fruits harm them, they need fruits more than other people, because their disease is caused by a lack of fruits.

I would like to refer to a case which is very painful for me to recall but has an important message. An acquaintance of mine, aged in his 30s who had an important post in a commercial company, developed heart disease. His heart and vessels didn't work sufficiently and his heartbeat was irregular because of a lack of expert cells. The doctors thought the only way to treat him was to send him to the USA to see a "famous" surgeon. This person tried live-food eating after reading my book. After 2-2.5 months, his heart recovered and the doctors were astonished. This patient was very glad of the result.

Sometime after he started to experience remedial reactions showing how his diet was helping him to get rid of the poisons in his body. But the people around him were skeptical about his decision to switch to live food eating and so called his doctor. It's clear that the doctor hadn't heard or read about remedial reactions and advised his patient not to eat anymore natural foods.

As a result of this the reactions stopped, and the patient seemed to improve and he gained 4-5 kilos of his weight, which he had lost during the live food eating period. For me, it was very clear that this temporary relief was the result of some months of live eating which would soon be destroyed and his health would deteriorate, as a result of switching to dead food eating. His family supported his decision as they couldn't see how a human could live on bunches of wheat, almonds, cucumber and tomato?!

One day he told me: "My family and I love our food and all we want to do is cook more 'delicious' food and eat as much as we can and enjoy it. We believe that this is the meaning of life."

And also his mother had said during his live-eating period: "I don't agree with this manner, why do you deprive yourself of these 'delicious' foods?! It's better to eat 'delicious' foods and die!" and this is what happened, he ate and died.

My wife, who is younger than me and wasn't gluttonous like me, but had countless maladies like heart disease, colds, angina, appendicitis, indigestion, unknown pains in her breasts and stomach and many other illnesses. She experienced some reactions like dizziness, foot pains and tumefaction and so on, which were like my reactions but a little less severe.

For a broad-minded person this is very easy to understand. Babies of dead food eaters are usually born with a weak body. Their mother's milk which is produced from dead foods is heavy and harmful. Babies' stomachs don't want to accept this harmful nutriment so they reject these foods and in doing so they can experience indigestion, lassitude, diarrhea, insomnia, perspiration or nervousness.

In this disorder, if a baby gets sick and had eaten some grapes and the skin happens to appear in his/her excretion, here the "sharp-sighted" doctor uncovers from his greatest "scientific knowledge", the cause of the sickness must be grapes and forbids eating grapes and all other live foods!

The conclusion of this process is clear; the baby becomes worse every day and hundreds of types of diseases such as gripe, angina, allergies, headaches, stomach aches, influenza, coughs, persistent fever and other issues are revealed one after another. In summary, all organs of the body work defectively because of the real hunger and lack of the main cells and casual microbes misuse from weakness of extra cells and sabotage in the body.

My children were always in this situation and we poor parents thought that in this "advanced" world with these "famous scientists", with these "equipped hospitals" and in these vast drugstores, a drug must certainly exist which could put an end to all these maladies and we just need to know the name of this miraculous drug and purchase it.

We visited doctor after doctor, from this city to that city, to find such a medicine.

In those sixteen years hundreds of medical tests had been taken, hundreds of different doctors, hundreds of types of medicine were tested and like a rule, always "strengthening food" like barbecue, chicken soup, liver, egg, milk, butter, had been prescribed.

First I travelled with my son to Paris and surrendered him to the famous American Hospital there.

But what could these "famous scientists" do for my children? Hundreds of intolerable medical tests had been carried out with more bills from the hospital, more dead food had been consumed and worse of all, hundreds of types of toxic drugs had been prescribed. In those days, cortisone and other terrible drugs (poisons) had been invented, so those doctors tried to test these poisons on my son, and in this situation, there was no discussion concerning natural and live foods. Today this ghastly situation continues in every hospital in the world.

I cannot forget those two memories at all, which remained in my mind forever.

In Paris, there was a shop selling fruit opposite one of the windows of our hotel which had excellent pears and peaches. My poor and weak son asked me to buy some pears and peaches for him, I didn't buy, but instead, chemical compotes had been entered in our home box by box. Another time, we had rented a garden in Vanak (an area in north of Tehran) to spend the summer. Boys pulled fresh and green walnuts from a great walnut tree. I had gotten money for each walnut and took them from babies to prevent them from eating these "harmful" walnuts.

My poor son perished under this tree from the real hunger.

Now some people ask me that how this son could remain alive for ten years without any natural food. I should say that of course that it's impossible to prevent a human from using natural foods completely. My children were occasionally eating an apple, an orange or a piece of watermelon and other fruits and also sometimes for the sake of not correctly baking foods, some cells hadn't been killed and their nutritive value had remained, but this very little amount of natural foods couldn't help their health and it only extended the pain.

When I lost my son, my daughter was eight years old. My son's symptoms were sometimes seen in her but a little milder. For the sake of fear that she would also befall her brother's destiny, I decided to take her abroad and prevent her from disease. I didn't know that I was entrusting my daughter to an executioner.

We took her to Hamburg and entrusted her to a famous hospital. They did all the medical tests they could, even cut a hole in her bones and extracted the marrow for medical tests, but they didn't find the cause of her disease. After that they became hopeless and handed my daughter over to a children's hospital where she saw a different doctor who was a wild and pitiless man. He started the medical tests which had been done before, but he didn't succeed in finding a reason for her disease and persistent fever.

When I carried my daughter to Hamburg, she was a weak child like thousands of other children and sometimes she had persistent fever about 37.5 degrees. But this pitiless doctor after two months conveyed my child to near death with his barbaric process. Each time he took blood from my child or was carrying out a boring medical test, my daughter's fever increased and as her fever increased, the amount of antibiotics was also increased, as he increased the antibiotics, her fever increased until finally it reached 41 degrees centigrade and after that it didn't decrease to less than 39 for several weeks. What was actually happening was that microbes, which reproduce every minute, fight against antibiotics and disregard them while poisons in the body's cells and their resistance against microbes decreases day by day.

I see that these tests harm my daughter, but what can I do? If I carry her to another hospital, these actions will be repeated again in there. I had this experience for twelve years. If I take her back to Tehran, I wondered what I had done for her.

This pitiless doctor didn't have any consideration. He treated my child like a laboratory animal and without heeding the questions of a father, increased the bill and completed his personal experiments, collected tens of mice and rabbits, took all of my daughter's blood and injected them and with foster microbes to try and recognize the type of microbe. This is "science", what can be said?!

Finally as a result of these poisonings, my daughter's kidneys became spoiled and she got persistent Nephritis. For me it was completely clear if my daughter had remained in Iran and her disease had developed gradually, like it had done in the past, perhaps it would never have been as bad after ten to fifteen years as it was when this pitiless man worsened it in two months.

Her sickness, which was a mystery for those European "scientists", today is very clear and easy for me to understand. The organs of my child didn't work properly because of lack of natural foods. And for the sake of impotent body cells, inner microbes always perform harmful acts and poisons which entered her body every day through dead foods and poisonous medicines, generating further poisoning. Nowadays also tens of thousands of children perish everyday because of this and no one even thinks of searching for the real agents of these hasty and inopportune deaths in medical sciences.

My daughter's health deteriorated to a point where the doctor told me she may only have one week to live if she stays as she is. He said: "The last cure is to get cortisone to her or cut a hole in her body and extract a piece of flesh and test it." I resisted against this work strongly. During this time, I found a German version of a book written by "Bircher Benner" which after reading it I felt like a lamp was shining in the darkness for me. However I learnt German for five months without a teacher, but I understood immediately that the reason for my children's diseases was unnatural feeding and using drugs.

I shared this matter with the doctor and forced him to accept the truth. He stopped using drugs and dead foods immediately and let us use natural and live foods. A sudden miracle appeared from the first day. Her fever decreased from 40-41 to 37.5 centigrade degrees, her eyes opened, my daughter sat up in bed, however she couldn't move before, and three days after live eating her status became much better.

As I saw this situation, I said to myself that we can feed the child at home better. So four days after starting live eating, we brought her into a room which we rented in a house. The amount of urine which was not more than 200 milliliters per day in hospital, at home increased to two liters per day, meaning ten times more! A few days later when the doctor knocked at the door of our room to meet my daughter, my daughter ran and opened the door and the doctor was very surprised.

This unjust doctor for the sake of fear lest we complain about his caddish and inhuman actions, didn't get my daughter's file to us containing his useless and inept reasons.

I took my daughter to the Bircher Benner clinic in Zurich and remained with her for twenty five days. Unfortunately Bircher Benner passed away before that and his children managed the sanatorium. There wasn't a complete 100% live eating there. They had a kitchen and they did serve live foods and didn't serve meats, but using dead foods, dairy and artificial vitamins were usual. In other words, it was only a vegetarian place.

The clinic did cause me to make a mistake. From that time, my personal reading about live eating started. Like Bircher Benner and others, I thought that we should use live eating temporarily and only for treatment. I believed that if I left the child to eat what she wanted, get her a little more fruits, feed her a little less meat and sometimes get her some chemical vitamin pills, all things will be returned back to normal. I didn't know yet that the artificial vitamin is a fatal poison like other drugs. For the sake of that my child seemed healthy when we arrived in Tehran and she swam and was going to school, I didn't understand that for all maladies especially for kidney diseases, we can trust only 100% live eating. After one or two years her kidneys sickened slowly and after four years I lost my daughter. Now my comfort is that I think perhaps God wanted this to happen to rescue millions of other children from death. I count those children as my children who grow with live eating in different parts of the world.

Now the time has come to notify everyone and get them to understand that approval and confirmation of dead foods and chemical materials to people especially forbidding them from using natural foods is the most terrible sin. These poor doctors don't know that with this antithetic process, they harm themselves and their children more than others."

Please note that remedial reactions are different in everyone and in some people, especially in older overweight people, severe pains may be experienced sometimes. These reactions are not dangerous, they are because of the natural cleansing of the body, but to relieve the intensity of pain, we can use some medical herbs. So if you feel bad, you can seek the advice of an experienced raw vegan or natural hygienist.

What is Cancer?

Cancer is one of the most dangerous diseases of our time and our many attempts to eradicate it have been unsuccessful.

Hovanessian's view on cancer

Arshavir Ter-Hovanessian writes about his view on the subject in another of his books, written in Persian, called: "**Cooked eating; a lethal habit**".

Despite more research being carried out on cancer since Hovanessian wrote the book, I think what Hovanessian found with his intuition is noteworthy because it led to good results. The section below is translated by me from his book (in Persian) and wherever the author's view was incomplete I've added footnotes:

"As I have written in the previous book (Raw-eating), the cooked food eater has two different bodies: the main body and the factitive body, containing the damaged and sick cells caused by eating unhealthy foods and storing poisons in the body.

The factitive body is nourished with dead foods[30]. Biologists try very much to recognize the difference between the natural cells and cancerous cells, and the only difference found so far is that cancerous cells have a very simple shape and they don't have any useful purpose[31]. The only purpose of these cells is to chase protein, devour it and reproduce[32]. As we know, the extra cells found in the bodies of dead food eaters have this exact feature, and only the slight difference between their extra cells and cancerous cells, means that the main body controls the extra cells to spread them to the empty parts of the body[33].

Both extra cells and cancerous cells are produced from baked and cooked foods. Extra cells aren't able to absorb the huge amount of unnatural foods completely, so a big part of it (dead food) fights with the defenses of the body and turns it to extra heat and disappears without any benefit. When one or more numbers of these cells succeed in finding independence, they start to devour extra foods, especially animal amino acids in an unbelievable manner. Thus, it starts from some little cells and grows into a monster (cancer) which frightens all us all.

A realistic person, who always engages his mind with important subjects, can't help but wonder how much time, energy and money scientists spend researching cures for cancer. They collect hundreds of kinds of carcinogenic material in their research, which aren't related to the main causes of cancer except nourishment.

Everybody should ask themselves: okay, we suppose that different poisons, body damages, scalding, viruses and other (harmful) things can prevent cells from carrying out their duties, damage them, devitalize and kill them. But which factor can give such power to a little (cancerous) cell so it can grow and reproduce so it harms the amazing formation of the body and eventually destroy it?

A person creates this power in their kitchen with the most severity! So, each piece of cooked food is carcinogenic, which means all pieces of unhealthy cooked foods produce cancer together.

Scientists find the main cause of cancer in their research several times. They find undeniable evidence, they even confirm it, but when the subject of changing food is considered, they escape from it! Why is this? Because they don't want to see or accept any unnatural thing in their eating habits, in particular they don't want to criticize bread, which people eat every day often as their main staple. They don't want to see that the natural bread is live wheat, and they waste it by skinning it, flouring it, leavening it and baking it.

Cell biologists observe that cancerous cells miss the special organs so they don't have the ability of do useful activities. By their view, the cells of the body in so-called healthy people were perfect and fault-free at first and after that, they lost their natural features and power due to some carcinogenic materials. (They don't know that there is not even one complete healthy person amongst cooked food eaters!). In other words faults in cells isn't related to any accidental factor except the food which humans eat every day. These people don't accept that a lot of dead, poisonous, worthless and hollow cells enter the body of dead food eaters every day.

Canadian American biologist Edmund Vincent Cowdry has collected all the evidence which scientists all over the world has gained during their research, and has published them in a book called Cancer cells. A realistic reader can easily understand that the main cause of cancer and its main factors are very clear. Here I quote some parts of this book for readers:

Cowdry writes: "with losing a part or all special organs in cancerous cells, their producing power decreases on the basis of its quantum. Doing duties isn't possible without the necessary organs.[34]"

Cowdry didn't know that cells need raw materials to build producer organs, and when raw foods turn into baked (dead) foods, neither suitable formation remains for cells to do any useful activity!

Cowdry adopts the Rusch method and writes: "Natural cells have machines and systems which determine their perfection. Operations of these machines maximizes when it reaches to a fixed ambit.[35]"

He goes on to write: "in the way of cancer, cells lose one or more of their activity abilities. It means that hereditary changes occur in them. They are compelled to lose one or more useful devices to reach independence. Semen and sperm are complete cells so they don't turn into cancer.[36]"

The most important action of cancerous cells is to hunt hydric stuff, devour animal protein, devour amino acids, and produce artificial proteins and much other desolation.

"Cancerous cells extract amino acids from the body's supply like a hydric trap and don't repay it.[37]" according to Cowdry, he continues: "it seems that hydric metabolism of cancerous cells in their process; try to steal the materials which the body's active cells need very much."

Cowdry believes that animal protein is very necessary for the body. Christensen and Handerson think that the predominance of cancerous cells in collecting amino acids and their immeasurable growth in a weak creature is an important factor[38]. As they thought, the weakening of the body was the result of animal protein shortage, not a lack of natural foods!

Cancerous cells synthesis protein constantly. Cowdry writes: "it has been seen sometimes that malign cancer grows with unnatural synthesis and even with producing unnatural protein. New proteins appear continuously for growth of cancerous tumor, in natural synthesis status it is controlling with disintegration, means in one side, new cells are producing and in another side, old cells die.[39]"

Then, Cowdry quotes from Gasperson: "it seems that there is a fundamental difference in protein producing system between malign cancerous cells and normal cells. In the cells of malign tumor, interceptor systems which usually determine some limits in actions of protein producing, stop in cancerous cells more or less.[40]"

Protein, and again, protein! Dear reader! This is the protein which doctors suggest everyone consumes. As you observe, these proteins and amino acids are useful for cancerous cells.

Cowdry confirms that: "the cells of the human body are small persons which are very complex and perhaps they are made from more than ten thousand different parts. Even recognition of the math formula of for-five synthesizers is a very difficult work, so, how we can trade with thousands of different organs?[41]" Yes, the biologists who know very little about formation and activity of a cell, define the destiny of people! They entrust calculations of the main engineer (the nature) to fire and they think they know how much fat, starch, protein and vitamins these cells need per day, and with their vain, wrong and dangerous calculations, devastate both their mind and the minds of people completely.

Many cell biologists have collected countless evidences which show that a reduction in the amount of food we eat helps to prevent the growth of cancer. In the period of World War, victims of cancer decreased in Denmark, Russia and Germany as a result of food rations.

According to the views of Hindhede polyphagia is very effective in cancer events. Cowdry gives examples from samples which are tested on animals.

Biochemist Clive Maine MacCay shows that limiting nourishment prevents cancer or decreases its growth speed.

The rate that cancer grows in experiments on mice depends on the amount of food they eat. McCay and his friends have researched mice which eat just enough to survive but not enough to grow. They observed one group of these mice which remained young for seven hundred days and preserved another group for nine hundred days and didn't let them reach maturity, however in normal situations, their longevity was six hundred days. When they got enough food again, these mice remained alive for more than one thousand and four hundred days, more than twice their normal longevity. The next evidence showed that in 198 mice which were fed with their "normal" diet, 150 cases of cancer were observed, while only 38 cases of cancerous tumors were seen in 200 mice which had only eaten little amounts of food .

They tried several times to find evidence from insurance offices to show what the relation between body weight and fatality is. 7,740,672 policies were checked. In each one hundred thousand documents, it showed 37 deaths for heavy weights more than normal, 32 for normal weight and 24 deaths for weights less than normal weight. A very noteworthy (but regretful) calculation for 50 years, from 1900 to 1950, symmetric with "development" of the medical sciences and growth fatalities of cancer and apoplexy is thus:

In this 50 year period, we have seen an increase from 64 to 139.6 deaths by cancer per one hundred thousand deaths. And also it went from 244 to 478.1 deaths from heart diseases (approximately double). More interesting than others, from 1950 to 1964 (a period of 14 years), it went from 139.6 to 151.3 deaths caused by cancer (per one hundred thousand people), and also death by heart diseases went from 478.1 to 508.6.

The American scientists get these documents from official offices of insurance companies. Cancer didn't occur among wild animals in their natural environment. After that they fed monkeys in captivity with unnatural foods for a long time, and one or two cancer-like tumors has been observed in them. In the depths of the oceans, where the destructive hand of humans hadn't yet reached, cancerous tumors are extremely rare.

Cowdry confirms that the quality of food is very effective in cancer. He writes: "finally, the truth shows outright that those animals who eat natural foods have less tendency to get cancer in comparison with those ones nourished by filtered foods."

The only great groups of creatures which are defended from cancer completely, live in the deep seas. This truth is more important when we know the populations of creatures in seas are three times more than on land. Now unfortunately "civilized" people pollute water of the seas, too.

Finally, during this search, biologists find the main factor of cancer. They see it, and even confirm it but ignore it with calmness and indifference, like the subject of action is another thing. Cowdry writes: *"the opinion which says that overuse or lack of some materials can cause cancer is accrediting slowly."*

They see the effects of natural foods and so Cowdry writes: "finally, the truth shows outright that those animals who nourish with the natural foods, have less tendency to cancer in comparison with those ones which are nourished by filtered foods." These filtered foods are formed from Casein, amyloid materials, cotton seeds oil, chemical vitamins and minerals.

Hovanessian continues:

"Cell biologists collect field mice from wild lands, which are protected against cancer (in their natural environment), and keep them in shelves, treat them like weak children and nourish them with "standard" foods, force them into sexual intercourse, protect them strongly and don't let them have contact with any carcinogen material whether chemical, physical or biological. But nevertheless, eighty percent of these mice get cancer with "spontaneously" and "unknown" reasons!

What a surprise that Cowdry doesn't see that it is the unnatural foods and unnatural environment which causes cancer, but nevertheless, he writes: *"in all cancerous tumors which doctors studied, maybe less than one percent of them have been in contact with these carcinogenic factors."*

But against it, we saw how unnatural foods made eighty cancerous mice from one hundred healthy mice. In another experiments, 150 mice got cancer from a total 198 mice! When reducing the amount of food this number (of cancerous mice) decreases from 150 to 38.

Now let's see what result the scientists have got from this valuable evidence:

Cowdry reached a surprising result, he says: "All of the research tested on animals, needs caution if we want to test them on humans. The human is an omnivorous creature who collects different foods from each part of the world, but other creatures eat local herbs. The lifespan of humans is much longer than laboratory animals. Thus, it is not possible to test this presumptive diet which takes a very long time to show the progress of cancer."

Mr. Cowdry and partners! You have found that natural foods prevent cancer. In other words, unnatural foods cause these dangerous diseases. Is there anything more important than cooking and baking which turns natural foods into unnatural stuffs?! Why do you continue your experiments and studies?! In fact, you found the main cause of the dangerous malady of cancer, what are you searching for, next?! Which more important factor than animal proteins and animal amino acids can create this satanic demon in the human body? This animal protein which you recommend to children, older people and sick people!

You find the main factor of cancer, so why you don't inform people of this very important news? Do you pity people that lest they remain deprived from the joy of baked foods?!

You are mistaken to think it takes 20-25 years to get cancer. No Mr. Cowdry! It only takes one second for a cell to dissever from its neighbor and change into a cancerous cell. Didn't you know a child which is born with cancer?! Didn't you see two-year-old cancerous kids?!

Be sure that if industries of baking and medicines of "civilized" people go forward with this speed, seventy percent of people will be born with cancer like laboratory mice several generations later. You report the truth, and let people decide themselves whether they want to nourish healthy with natural foods or perish by unnatural and dangerous foods.

This is amazing. See how these biologists and doctors have been perverted as much as they didn't understand yet that cooking and baking is a very dangerous factor which disarranges natural laws and causes all misfortunes of people. Cowdry has taken what he has searched for, and he continues his search in the darkness still. Now everyone in the world knows about the harm caused by cigarettes. Cigarette contains a poison called "nicotine", but this poison can't produce cells. It's protein in meat and dairy products which can produce cells. When the body is producing cancer, it searches for a weak and appropriate point to start this work. The lung, which has weakened by the negative effects of nicotine, is a suitable point for cancer to grow. Sometimes a part of the hand or leg collide with another thing and ulcerates, this wound isn't treated and turns into cancer.

I had some glandular things in some parts of my body. For example, under the skin of my testicles there had been hidden a gland as big as a pea, which has shrunk after starting raw eating. Eventually when I pressed it, a piece of dead and black flesh erupted. Also, I had two small wounds in my fingers which weren't treated for several years. It was clear that these were alien fleshes which has remained for some time and didn't want to connect with the flesh of body. I have observed how these alien fleshes were growing slowly and eat my body. After raw-eating, it stopped for some years, solved in my body and disappeared.

Cowdry got evidence from the archives of the American courts which shows that workers who had an ulcerated leg or hand during their work in factory and didn't treat it, it often turned into cancer. The courts counted these small wounds as the main factor of death and has condemned the owner of factory to pay blood money. There are countless such trials in documents of these courts."

National Cancer Institute's view

Referring to content on the website of the National Cancer Institute (NCI)[42] we see a similar view in some points about cancerous cells however they don't give us a good explanation of the main causes of cancer. In the section Defining Cancer on the NCI website, it says:

"Cancer is a term used for diseases in which abnormal cells divide without control and are able to invade other tissues. Cancer cells can spread to other parts of the body through the blood and lymph system.

Cancer is not just one disease but many diseases. There are more than 100 different types of cancer. Most cancers are named for the organ or type of cell in which they start - for example, cancer that begins in the colon is called colon cancer.

All cancers begin in cells, the body's basic unit of life. To understand cancer, it's helpful to know what happens when normal cells become cancer cells.

The body is made up of many types of cells. These cells grow and divide in a controlled way to produce more cells as they are needed to keep the body healthy. When cells become old or damaged, they die and are replaced with new cells.

However, sometimes this orderly process goes wrong. The genetic material (**DNA**) of a cell can become damaged or changed, producing **mutations** that affect normal cell growth and division. When this happens, cells do not die when they should and new cells form when the body does not need them. The extra cells may form a mass of tissue called a **tumor**."

Origins of Cancer

Dr. Otto Heinrich Warburg who was awarded the Nobel Prize in Physiology in 1931, wrote this about cancer[43]:

"Cancer, above all other diseases, has countless secondary causes. Almost anything can cause cancer. But, even for cancer, there is only one prime cause. The prime cause of cancer is the replacement of the respiration of oxygen (oxidation of sugar) in normal body cells by fermentation of sugar.

All normal body cells meet their energy needs by respiration of oxygen, whereas cancer cells meet their energy needs in great part by fermentation. All normal body cells are thus obligate aerobes, whereas all cancer cells are partial anaerobes. From the standpoint of the physics and chemistry of life this difference between normal and cancer cells is so great that one can scarcely picture a greater difference. Oxygen gas, the donor of energy in plants and animals, is dethroned in the cancer cells and replaced by the energy yielding reaction of the lowest living forms, namely the fermentation of sugar.

In every case, during the cancer development, the oxygen respiration always falls, fermentation appears, and the highly differentiated cells are transformed into fermenting anaerobes, which have lost all their body functions and retain only the now useless property of growth and replication. Thus, when respiration disappears, life does not disappear, but the meaning of life disappears, and what remains are growing machines that destroy the body in which they grow.

All carcinogens impair respiration directly or indirectly by deranging capillary circulation, a statement that is proven by the fact that no cancer cell exists without exhibiting impaired respiration. Of course, respiration cannot be repaired if it is impaired at the same time by a carcinogen.

To prevent cancer it is therefore proposed first to keep the speed of the blood stream so high that the venous blood still contains sufficient oxygen; second, to keep high the concentration of hemoglobin in the blood; third, to add always to the food, even of healthy people, the active groups of the respiratory enzymes; and to increase the doses of these groups, if a precancerous state has already developed. If at the same time exogenous carcinogens are excluded rigorously, then much of the endogenous cancer may be prevented today."

Preventing disease

There are different factors which contribute to the causes of cancer. We must aim to avoid all toxins like tobacco and alcohol as much as possible. But changing our diet is the easiest thing that we can do to prevent cancer.

The necessity of using natural food to remain healthy is very clear, if not, cells of the body get damaged more and more until the foods aren't natural and healthy. So, the best way to prevent and eradicate cancer (and also other diseases) is to follow a natural diet like raw veganism.

In her book *'Life without Cancer: How to Stop Making Disease in Your Body'* Andrea Lambert[44] looks at the root cause of cancer, the triggers that can cause it. Lambert educates us about listening to our body's needs so we can prevent disease and live a healthy life.

"One of the most important concepts I have learned during my journey is simply called The Seven Stages of Disease. This is a fascinating Naturopathic concept that offers us the ability to "hear" what our body needs. According to this concept, there is only one disease. When we break that word down and say it in syllables, Dis-ease, that's really what it's all about, the lack of ease in the body. This is a clue![45]

The stages of disease are as follows[46]:

Stage 1: Enervation (lack of sleep or adequate rest)
Stage 2: Toxemia (excessive toxins)
Stage 3: Irritation (constant toxic exposure to the same area)
Stage 4: Inflammation (swelling in over-irritated areas)
Stage 5: Ulceration (holes to drain excessive toxins)
Stage 6: Induration (tumor formation)
Stage 7: Cancer (anaerobic cell formation)"

"Deprive a cell 35% of its oxygen for 48 hours and it may become cancerous." Dr. Warburg has made it clear that the root cause of cancer is oxygen deficiency, which creates an acidic state in the human body. He also discovered that cancer cells are anaerobic and can't survive in the presence of high levels of oxygen, as found in an alkaline state.[47]

The amount and types of toxicity will affect the body in different ways. Toxins, such as trans-fats, coat the cells blocking the cell receptors creating a situation where oxygen and nutrients cannot enter the cell as easily. Waste cannot be removed from the cell as easily either. This means the life giving cellular respiration can't happen. An analogy would be overexerting us during a cardio workout. This can leave you feeling sore the next day due to lactic acid build up from not getting enough oxygen to your cells. Our cells will switch to anaerobic respiration which means chemical reactions without oxygen take place leaving lactic acid as a byproduct. This acid makes our muscles feel sore. This is a mild example of lack of oxygen for a short amount of time that is quickly reversed when we stop. Please don't use this as an excuse to not exercise but maybe to exercise a little more gently.

Cancer cells are primitive cells. They are triggered to grow from lack of oxygen to the healthy cells. These primitive cells are disconnected from the normal communication system and end up doing their own thing to survive. They need a lot more fuel, due to their simplified mechanism and primitive inefficiency; therefore, they will consume many more times the fuel (glucose & fructose) you put into your body leaving you feeling weak. Your healthy cells get the leftovers. If you don't change your diet, the glucose you consume will feed the cells first and the fructose you consume will allow for faster cell division, leading to faster cancer spreading throughout the body. They want to survive too and are programmed to multiply fast without the typical cell death codes (apoptosis) a normal cell has.[48]"

Protein

Many meat eaters were once afraid to go vegetarian as they were concerned about their protein intake if they were to make the change. However, it's a false belief that protein only exists in meat, eggs and animal products or that the human body cannot absorb plant protein as well. Today, it is widely accepted that a healthy vegan diet contains sufficient protein to satisfy our requirements.

In the late nineteenth century people believed that the human body required 145 grams of protein every day, while today this figure has been reduced to 50 or even 40 grams per day[49].

As a general rule, between 10 percent and 15 percent of your total calories should come from protein. So if you consume 2,000 calories per day, at least 200 should come from protein, or about 50 grams. You should try to eat around one gram of protein per one kilogram of body weight, or around 0.4 grams per pound.

The truth is that protein exists in all foods and all plants or more precisely in all cells. Even in one large orange there contains about six to nine percent protein (by calorie) and plant protein is purer and healthier than animal protein, which is full of bad cholesterol, saturated fats and hormones and can be polluted by many other poisons and bacteria. Fruits and vegetables contain useful chemicals like antioxidants which are vital for the body. Plants like lentils, seaweed, broccoli and some beans have more protein per calorie than meat[50]. What is important to note is that our bodies do not require a large amount of protein as an excess of it can be harmful[51].

Protein requirements differ depending on body size and daily activity, for example athletes need a little more protein[52]. However, some researchers do not agree with this statement and say that even athletes do not need much more protein than non athletes[53]. Fortunately no issues arise if you are satisfying your protein needs with a natural diet and raw veganism can be far better for athletes.

We know that the biggest and most powerful animals such as elephants, giraffes, horses and buffalo are herbivores. Also monkeys, which have the most similarities to humans are herbivores (frugivores) and are very powerful animals; so if plant proteins are not satisfactory to some people, why don't these animals suffer from a lack of protein?

Protein is one important prerequisite to produce any cell, so there is no plant or animal without protein. Some people believe that meats make man strong but the idea of becoming strong by eating flesh is a very droll delusion. In the wild carnivores are often no stronger than an equal sized herbivore animal. Carnivores often attack in groups because they are not strong enough to fight big animals alone.

Meat is not useful for the human body just as it is not useful for other herbivores, for example if we feed a cow with meat powder it will get mad cow disease[54].

It is very clear that meat consumption for humans can cause different diseases, whether it is heart problems, cancer or even impotence[55]. Even the bodies of athletes wear out sooner if they consume meat which can lead to strokes or cancer. So there is really no hope for people who don't exercise regularly and also eat unhealthy food.

I was told many times as a child that: "if you don't eat flesh, you will become weak"; a myth which is laughable for an experienced vegetarian person. However, in unhealthy vegetarians different deficiencies are observed such as iron deficiency, but a lack of protein is something that vegetarians do not suffer until there is another health problem like digestive and pancreatic disorder. A healthy and balanced lifestyle shouldn't lead to any digestive issues.

Protein in mothers' milk

On the basis of different medical experiences the rate of protein in a mother's milk is about 1-2 percent by weight or about 5-10 percent by calorie[56]. Even with such a low rate of protein this is enough to ensure the fast healthy growth of an infant and therefore for each animal, there is no milk better than the milk of a mother because the nutritive particles are an exact fit for her baby's needs.

There doesn't seem to be a definitive reason why the percentage of protein differs but it may be because the growth rate of a baby is different during each period of formation, so his/her needs are different at each stage. We know that the speed of growth is very fast in the first few months, so the baby needs more protein during this time. From this I would say the rate of protein required for the human body is about 1-2 percent by weight or 5-10 percent by calorie.

What is interesting to note is that sweet fruits and also many vegetables have a similar rate of protein to mothers' milk as they mostly contain the same amount of protein compared to breast milk[57]. This is another example to support the view that humans are naturally frugivores, not omnivores.

It's not necessary to eat dairy or cereals to make up for the fact you have eliminated meat from your diet. As humans we don't need to eat meat at all, so it is meaningless to search for a meat substitution.

Tailoring our diet around our nutritional needs is vital to remain healthy and each essential nutrient for the body, which does not include uric acid, excess hormones or saturated animal fats, should be consumed in the right amounts. A lack of these nutrients is harmful as is an exorbitance of these nutrients.

Some vegetables like broccoli and also most fatty fruits (such as avocado) as well as nuts and seeds, contain more protein than red meat, while they don't have high amounts of uric acid, saturated fats and other poisons which are found in animal flesh. So consuming these high protein plants in small amounts is recommended.

Protein deficiency

A lack of protein can lead to different diseases. The warning signs are often hard cavities, brittle nails, exorbitant emaciation and skin problems. Other signs of a minor protein deficiency can take months or years to develop. They might include blood sugar instability, muscle or joint pain and general feelings of weakness or fatigue[58]. A severe lack of protein can be fatal.

A severe lack of protein occurs due to the following reasons:

If there is absolutely nothing to eat such as in some African countries where thousands of people perish because of hunger and malnutrition every year. In these countries, even those people who have food to eat are still perishing from different maladies, because their food is unhealthy and very poor in nutritional value, particularly in minerals and vitamins.

Some diseases like pancreatic cancer or hard digestive problems can prevent the absorption of protein while diseases like kidney disease can cause too much protein to be expelled from the body so that even if you over consume protein to compensate it doesn't help.

According to the article: "*Plant-Based Diets Are Not Nutritionally Deficient*" from the website of the Natural Institutes of Health[59], the vegetarian myths which concern people are not scientifically true. The article explains why a plant-based diet is a healthy option:

"The risks are so low that illnesses because of the lack of any of these essential nutrients, including protein, have not been reported to occur on any natural human diet (as long as calorie intake is sufficient). Dietary manipulation or supplementation to improve the overall quality, or to increase the absolute quantity, of protein, iron, calcium, or fatty acids has not been found to be beneficial. To the contrary, excess protein is a major contributor to bone loss."

What isn't yet clear is whether cooked proteins are just as beneficial as raw proteins. There are many controversies surrounding this matter but I will go as far to say that most denatured proteins or those proteins which are altered or destroyed by the cooking process are not better than their raw state, similar to other nutrients in foods which are destroyed by cooking at high temperatures[60].

Too much protein could be dangerous

The human body has its own recycling system so valuable matter contained in our cells is recycled to make new cells. This natural recycling process is very exact and with the least possible losses if the body remains in a healthy state, so the body needs very little amounts of protein, despite what many people think. This logical idea is supported with several scientific studies[61].

We do not need too much protein every day; we don't even need to eat food every day, as we see in nature all animals fast at some point throughout the year[62], whether it is through hibernation or aestivation, which helps their body to cleanse itself.

Fasting is also helpful for the human body and is only really useful when we don't re-pollute it with dead foods after. But an excess amount of protein can be harmful and can cause an increase in blood acidity which can lead to kidney stones, osteoporosis and even cancer[63].

Are plant-based proteins defective?

The "incomplete protein" myth was inadvertently promoted by the 1971 book: 'Diet for a Small Planet', by Frances Moore Lappe. In it, the author stated that plant foods do not contain all the essential amino acids, so in order to be a healthy vegetarian, you needed to eat a combination of certain plant foods in order to get all of the essential amino acids; a theory known as "complementary protein", which has since been proven to be untrue.[64]

The complementary protein myth[65]

One of the sources of the protein combining myth was a book called: 'Diet for a Small Planet', published in 1971. The author, Frances Moore-Lappé, wanted to promote meatless eating because meat production wastes a large amount of resources. But she knew her readers would think you couldn't get enough protein on a vegetarian diet, so she set out to reassure them, by telling them that if they carefully combined various plant foods, like rice and beans, the inferior plant proteins would become just as "complete" as the ones in meat.

Lappé got her idea from studies that were done 100 years ago, on rats. The researchers found that rats grew best when the proteins in their diets were in the same proportion as those found in animal foods. From this finding, animal proteins were arbitrarily labeled first-class while plant proteins were deemed inferior. The problem with this conclusion is that rats are not humans; baby rats actually need a higher percentage of protein than baby humans because they grow a lot faster. People grow slowly. It takes a baby half a year to double its birth weight whereas a rat does this in only four and a half days. So clearly rats are going to need more protein. In fact, rats' milk contains 49% protein (by calorie), much higher than the mere 6% found in human mother's milk.

Also another comparison between the milk of humans and that of rats show this obvious difference very well; protein is only about 1.3 percent of human milk by weight, while the milk of rats contains about 8.4 percent protein. If ablactated rats are fed only with human milk, they will not have proportional growth. The World Health Organization (WHO) has since abandoned this incompatible method for evaluating proteins for the human body.

But it wasn't long before Lappé realized her mistake. In the 1981 edition of her book: '*Diet for a Small Planet*', she recanted:

"In 1971 I stressed protein complementing because I assumed that the only way to get enough protein ... was to create a protein as usable by the body as animal protein. In combating the myth that meat is the only way to get high-quality protein, I reinforced another myth. I gave the impression that in order to get enough protein without meat, considerable care was needed in choosing foods. Actually, it is much easier than I thought."

Essential Amino Acids

In 1952 William Rose and his colleagues completed research that determined the human requirements for the eight essential amino acids. They set the minimum amino acid requirement by making it equal to the greatest amount required by any single person in their study. To set the recommended amino acid requirement, they simply doubled the minimum requirements. This "recommended amino acid requirement" was considered a "definitely safe intake."

Today, if you calculate the amount of each essential amino acid provided by unprocessed plant foods and compare these values with those determined by Rose, you will find that any single one, or combination, of these whole natural plant foods provides all of the essential amino acids. Furthermore, these whole natural plant foods provide not just the minimum requirements but provide amounts far greater than the recommended requirements.

Modern researchers know that it is virtually impossible to design a calorie-sufficient diet based on unprocessed whole natural plant foods that is deficient in any of the amino acids.[66]

A fruit-based raw vegan diet which includes nuts, fatty fruits, seeds and vegetables is very rich in all nutrients and supplies all of our body's needs[67].

Science and experiences show clearly that a natural diet poses no risk to the human body. As a vegetarian athlete Fauja Singh is a successful marathon runner who, now more than 100-years-old and a world record breaker, is a perfect example of how athletes do not need to eat flesh to be strong.

To be a strong healthy individual you need to exercise regularly and follow a healthy diet that does not include the consumption of dead flesh.

Calcium, healthy bones and the milk paradox

I had a lot of worries when I first became a vegan, but I continued to research the subject and sought information from other vegans. I discovered more facts which amazed me, such as the theory that our body cannot absorb calcium from dairy products and in some cases is forced to take calcium from our bones.[68] The excess animal protein and sodium found in cow's milk leeches calcium from the bones, causing severe bone deterioration[69].

Milk and other animal products acidify the pH balance in our body. In correcting this our body draws the calcium from our bones as calcium is an acid neutralizer thus weakening our bones.

Countries which have the highest rate of milk and dairy consumption such as the USA, the UK and Scandinavian countries, also have the highest rate of osteoporosis. However the statistics may not be very accurate as they don't consider all variable situations, for example in this case, a lack of sunlight in some countries can contribute to osteoporosis. In his article *'Got Milk? You Don't Need It'* Mark Bittman talks about why we don't need cow's milk and the effects it can have on our bodies:

http://opinionator.blogs.nytimes.com/2012/07/07/got-milk-you-dont-need-it/

Calcium is not the only mineral that our bones need. Some other vital minerals and vitamins are needed for bones such as magnesium, vitamin D and vitamin K[70].

Homogenized milk

Homogenization is a process that some natural healing enthusiasts refer to as "the worst thing that dairymen did to milk." The homogenization process, to stop the fat separating from the milk, involves pushing it through a fine filter at pressures of around 4,000 pounds per square inch. The purpose is to reduce the size of the fat globules so it no longer separates. The fat molecules are then able to disperse more easily throughout the milk, which prevents the "creaming" or thickening of the milk. It is these fat molecules that become harmful for the body because they enter into our arteries and can cause heart problems.

Homogenized milk bypasses the normal digestive processes and delivers steroid and protein hormones to the human body both from the cow and the artificial ones which have been injected into the animal to produce more milk.

Proteins were created to be easily broken down by the digestive system. Homogenization disrupts this and ensures their survival so that they enter the bloodstream. Many times the body reacts to foreign proteins by producing histamines, and then mucus. Sometimes homogenized milk proteins resemble a human protein and can become triggers for autoimmune diseases such as diabetes, multiple sclerosis, cancer and heart disease.

When we eat or drink foods that have been pasteurized and homogenized, the increase in unusable proteins forces the body to quickly use up many enzymes and other vital nutrients to process it. Pasteurized milk can also lead to nutritional deficiencies. Protein, fat and sugar particles in denatured milk easily pass through the intestinal lining and often cause inflammation and allergic reactions.[71]

Why cow milk is not good for us?

When anyone states that cow's milk is harmful for the body, the general consensus is that milk provides us with calcium and essential nutrients. But to this I question whether the person is a calf or a baby? Think about it this way: a child feeding from their mothers past a certain age is often frowned upon yet adults drink gallons of milk…although not from their mommies, but from cows. Does this make sense to you? It certainly doesn't to me.

While breast milk is so vital and changes with the baby's needs, cow's milk was only meant for calves. When a (human) mother first starts a nursing session, her baby gets foremilk, which is lower in fat and higher in lactose, a milk sugar that is important for the baby's development. As the feeding progresses, the mother produces hind milk which is higher in fat, so it helps baby feel full for longer.

According to renowned researcher and professor emeritus of nutritional biochemistry at Cornell University, Dr. T. Colin Campbell[72], casein, a protein which makes up a high percentage of the proteins found in cow's milk, is the "number one carcinogen [cancer-causing substance] that people come into contact with on a daily basis."

Most cow's milk has measurable quantities of herbicides, pesticides, dioxins (up to 200 times the safe levels), up to 52 powerful antibiotics (perhaps 53, with LS-50), blood, pus, feces, bacteria and viruses. Cow's milk can have traces of anything the cow ate including such things as radioactive fallout from nuke testing (the 50's strontium-90 problem)[73].

Risks of drinking cow's milk

The disadvantages of drinking milk are not a new discovery. Even in the articles which support the idea that milk is useful for bone health because of its high amounts of calcium (which is a paradox) many still refer to the dangers of cow's milk for human health, as it can increase the risk of prostate cancer and heart disease. This article that appeared on the Harvard School of Public Health website is an example of this:

http://www.hsph.harvard.edu/nutritionsource/calcium-full-story/

The following statements, which also show the disadvantages of drinking milk, have been taken from scientific research reports:

"Dairy products may play a major role in the development of allergies, asthma, sleep difficulties, and migraine headaches."
Israel Journal of Medical Sciences 1983; 19(9):806-809 Pediatrics 1989; 84(4):595-603

"In reality, cow's milk, especially processed cow's milk, has been linked to a variety of health problems, including: mucus production, hemoglobin loss, childhood diabetes, heart disease, atherosclerosis, arthritis, kidney stones, mood swings, depression, irritability, allergies."
Townsend Medical Letter, May, 1995, Julie Klotter, MD

"At least 50% of all children in the United States are allergic to cow's milk, many undiagnosed. Dairy products are the leading cause of food allergy, often revealed by diarrhea, constipation, and fatigue. Many cases of asthma and sinus infections are reported to be relieved and even eliminated by cutting out dairy."
Natural Health, July, 1994, Nathaniel Mead, MD

Milk: A-Z by Robert Cohen

The website: *www.NotMilk.com* has useful information about the dangers of milk, thanks to the endeavors of Robert Cohen. It contains an A-Z summary about cow's milk based on information from scientific journals. I have included it to show the importance of this issue.

Milk: A-Z

A is for Allergies

"In reality, cow's milk, especially processed cow's milk, has been linked to a variety of health problems, including: mucus production, hemoglobin loss, childhood diabetes, heart disease, atherosclerosis, arthritis, kidney stones, mood swings, depression, irritability, and allergies."
Townsend Medical Letter, May, 1995

B is for Breast Cancer

"Insulin-like growth factor-I (IGF-I, a cow's milk hormone) produces a 10-fold increases in RNA levels of cancer cells. IGF-I appears to be a critical component in cellular proliferation."
X.S.Li, Exp-Cell-Res., March 1994, 211 (1)

C is for Crohn's disease

"Mycobacterium paratuberculosis (bacteria not killed by Pasteurization) RNA was found in 100% of Crohn's diseases patients, compared with 0% of controls."
D. Mishina, Proceedings National Academy of Sciences USA:93: September, 1996

D is for Diabetes

"These new studies, and more than 20 well-documented previous ones, have prompted one researcher to say the link between milk and juvenile diabetes is 'very solid'."
Diabetes Care, 1994; 17 (12)

E is for Ear infections

"Milk allergies are very common in children. They are the leading cause of the chronic ear infections that plague up to 40% of all children under the age of six."
Julian Whitaker, M.D., "Health and Healing", October 1998, Volume 8, No. 10

F is for Fat

"Preference for a diet high in animal fat could be a pathogenic factor, and milk and high fat dairy products contribute considerably to dietary fat intake."
J. Am Coll Nutr, 2000 Apr, 19:2 Suppl.

G is for Growth factor

"The insulin-like growth factor (IGF) system is widely involved in human carcinogenesis. A significant association between high circulating IGF-I concentrations and an increased risk of lung, colon, prostate and pre-menopausal breast cancer has recently been reported."
International J Cancer, 2000 Aug, 87:4

H is for Heart disease

"For ischemic heart disease, milk carbohydrates were found to have the highest statistical association for males aged 35+ and females 65+. In the case of coronary heart disease, non-fat milk was found to have the highest association for males aged 45+ and females aged 75+, while for females 65-74, milk carbohydrates…had the highest associations."
Altern Med Rev, Aug 3, 1998

I is for Iron deficiency

"Cow's milk-induced intestinal bleeding is a well-recognized cause of rectal bleeding in infancy. In all cases, bleeding is resolved completely after instituting a cow's milk-free diet."
J Pediatr Surg, 1999 October, 34:10

J is for Juvenile illnesses

"At least 50% of all 11-year-old children in the United States are allergic to milk, many undiagnosed. Dairy products are the leading cause of food allergies, often revealed by constipation, diarrhea and fatigue. Asthma and sinus infections are reported to be eliminated by cutting out dairy."
Natural Health, July 1994, Frank Oski, M.D.

K is for Killer bacteria

"… curing alone may not be a sufficient pathogen control step to eliminate Salmonella, Listeria, and E. Coli 0157:H7 from Cheese."
J Food Prot, 1998 Oct, 61:10

L is for Lactose intolerance

"Lactose malabsorption and lactase deficiency are chronic organic pathogenic conditions characterized by abdominal pain and distention, flatulence, and the passage of loose, watery stools. Once correct diagnosis is established, the introduction of a lactose-free dietary regime relieves symptoms in most patients."
J Clin Gastroenterol, 1999 Apr, 28:3

M is for Mad cow disease

"A 24-year-old vegetarian has been diagnosed with Cruetzfeld-Jacob disease (the human form of mad cow disease). Scientists fear that milk and cheese may be the source of infection."
London Times, August 23, 1997

N is for Nasal congestion

"Symptoms of a milk-protein allergy include coughing, choking, gasping, nose colds, asthma and sneezing attacks…"
Annals of Allergy, 1951; 9

O is for Osteoporosis

"Osteoporosis is caused by a number of things, one of the most important being too much dietary protein."
Science, 1986, 233

P is for Pesticides and Pollution

"The level of dioxin in a single serving of Ben & Jerry's World's best vanilla Ice Cream tested was almost 200 times greater than the 'virtually [safe] dairy dose' determined by the USA Environmental Protection Agency."
Steve Milloy, author of junkscience.com (Milloy tested samples of ice cream for dioxins. The only major newspaper to report the story was the Detroit Free Press.), 11/8/99

Q is for Quixote syndrome

"I have two lasting impressions. One is that underestimating Robert Cohen's ability to damage the dairy industry is a big mistake. The other is a profound wish that the man was on our side."
Editorial by Teresa VanWagner, American Dairy Farm Magazine, Oct. 1998

R is for Rheumatoid Arthritis

"In the case of an eight-year-old female subject, juvenile rheumatoid arthritis was a milk allergy. After avoiding dairy products, all pain was gone in three weeks."
Journal of the Royal Society of Medicine, 1985, 78

S is for sudden infant death

"Those who consumed cow's milk were fourteen times more likely to die from diarrhea-related complications and four times more likely to die for pneumonia than were breast-fed babies. Intolerance to cow's milk products is a factor in sudden infant death syndrome."
The Lancet, vol.344, November 5, 1994

T is for Tuberculosis

"Diseases such as tuberculosis are transmissible by milk products."
Journal of Dairy Science, 1988; 71

U is for Uterine and Ovarian Cancer

"The uterus and ovary, like the breast, are hormone-sensitive organs. Not surprisingly, uterine and ovarian cancers are both linked to fatty diets in epidemiologic studies."
Cancer, 1966 ; 19

V is for Vitamin D-efficiency

"Exposure to sunlight provides most humans with their vitamin D requirement."
Journal of Nutrition, 1966 ; 126(4 Suppl.)

W is for WISCOWSINITIS

"These dairy men are organized, they're adamant, and they're massing an enormous amount of money that they're going to put into political activities, very frankly."
Secretary of the Treasury John Connally to President Richard Nixon, from the Watergate Tapes, March 23, 1971 (after president Nixon had received $3 million cash gift from dairy industry representatives in the oval office.)

X is for Xanthene oxidase

"Bovine milk xanthene oxidase (BMXO) may be absorbed and may enter the cardiovascular system. People with clinical signs of atherosclerosis have greater quantities of BMXO antibodies. BMXO antibodies are found in greater quantities in those patients who consume the largest volumes of homogenized milk and milk products."
The X-O Factor, by Kurt Oster, M.D., and Donald Ross, Ph.D.

Y is for Yin/Yang

"Scientific data suggest positive relationships between a vegetarian diet and a reduced risk of several chronic degenerative diseases and conditions, including obesity, coronary artery disease, hypertension, diabetes mellitus, and some types of cancer."
Journal of the American Dietetic Association, November 1997

Z is for Zits (Acne)

"We studied effects of growth hormone (GH) and insulin-like growth factors (IGFs), alone and with androgen, on sebaceous epithelial cell growth...IGF-I was the most potent stimulus of DNA synthesis. These data are consistent with the concept that increases in GH and IGF production contribute in complementary ways to the increase in sebum production during puberty."

Endocrinology, 1999 Sep, 140:9, 4089-94

We cannot even use milk in its natural state

Milk is a fluid which becomes toxic as soon as it comes into contact with air. In nature, the newborn takes milk directly from the breast of its mother without the milk being exposed to air. So the artificial process of getting milk from animals, putting it in different containers and transporting it to other places, is very harmful.

To ensure a cow's milk is fit for human consumption it has to be heated because of the different deadly bacteria it contains, like Malta fever[74], but if we heat it, its vitamins are destroyed and the proteins lose their nutritional value.

Turning milk into other fermented forms like yoghurt or cheese, is even more harmful. In my opinion cheese is one of the worst and unhealthiest foods as it contains too much salt.

The lactic acid in yoghurt uses up the oxygen in our blood making us feel sleepy. Too much lactic acid in the body can also lead to cancer[75]. Healthy food should give you energy, not waste your energy.

Eating dairy products can cause bad breath because of our inability to break down the lactose protein that's in dairy foods. This results in a buildup of amino acids, which then convert into volatile sulfur compounds due to anaerobic bacteria on the tongue[76]. Our tongue, teeth and palate are coated with millions of bacteria. After a drink of milk, these microbes go to work digesting the leftover lactose, lipids and proteins that coat the mouth. Over time, this digestive process results in an excess of hydrogen sulfide in the mouth, which causes a sour smell. Lactose intolerance may also cause halitosis. Experts recently wrote in the Chicago Tribune that while there are few medical studies linking lactose intolerance to bad breath, it was still a possibility[77].

Dairy causes many problems as not only is it a protein source for bad breath bacteria but it thickens nasal mucus making it harder to clear away. Of all the dairy products, cheese is the worst offender followed closely by milk[78].

Osteoporosis

"Osteoporosis is caused by a number of things, one of the most important being too much dietary protein." Science 1986; 233(4763)[79]

"Countries with the highest rates of osteoporosis, such as the United States, England, and Sweden, consume the most milk. China and Japan, where people eat much less protein and dairy food, have low rates of osteoporosis."
Nutrition Action Health letter, June, 1993

"Dietary protein increases the production of acid in the blood which can be neutralized by calcium mobilized from the skeleton."
American Journal of Clinical Nutrition, 1995; 61 (4)

"Even when eating 1400 mg of calcium daily, one can lose up to 4% of his or her bone mass each year while consuming a high-protein diet." American Journal of Clinical Nutrition 1979; 32(4)

"Increasing one's protein intake by 100% may cause calcium loss to double."
Journal of Nutrition, 1981; 111 (3)

"Consumption of dairy products, particularly over 20 years were associated with an increased risk of hip fractures…metabolism of dietary protein causes increased urinary excretion of calcium."
American Journal of Epidemiology 1994; 139

Calcium sources in plants

Calcium exists in many plant sources such as dark leafy green vegetables, sesame seeds, almonds, oranges and broccoli and do not make blood acidic, so the body can absorb plant-based calcium effectively.

Included are some examples of the amount of calcium in certain fruits and vegetables:

2 medium raw carrots contain about 40 milligrams (mg) of calcium.

10 dried figs contain 140 mg of calcium.

A medium naval orange contains about 60 mg of calcium.

2/3 cup of raisins contains about 53 mg of calcium.

100 grams broccoli contains about 47 mg of calcium.

100 grams almonds contain about 264 mg of calcium.

Reducing calcium loss

A number of factors affect calcium loss:

Diets that are high in protein cause more calcium to be lost through the urine. Protein from animal products is much more likely to cause calcium loss than protein from plant foods. This may be one reason that vegetarians tend to have stronger bones than meat-eaters.
Diets high in sodium increase calcium loss through urine.
Caffeine (in tea and coffee) increases the rate at which calcium is lost through urine.
Smoking increases the loss of calcium from the body.

A number of factors help to strengthen our bones such as:
Exercise, which is one of the most important factors in maintaining bone health.
Exposure to sunlight allows the body to make the bone-building hormone vitamin D.
Eating a plentiful amount of fruit and vegetables helps to restrict calcium loss.
Consuming calcium from plant-based sources, especially green vegetables provides one of the main building blocks for strengthening our bones[80].

Alternatives to cow milk

Fortunately there are alternatives to help wean us off cow's milk. Almond milk and soy milk does not contain any of the harmful ingredients found in cow's milk.

What should be noted is that soy milk has a high level of protein and too much is not good for you. Soy can be harmful especially for children and people with thyroid disorders. Personally, I don't use soy and recommend avoiding it as much as possible.

Some good substitutes for cow's milk are:

Almond milk: made from soaked and blended almonds or other nuts, such as cashew milk. It has a creamy consistency similar to a thick soy milk and a nutty taste perfect for making vegan fruit smoothies or other creamy drinks and desserts.

Raw and fresh coconut milk

Rice milk which is not as thick as soy or dairy milk, and has a somewhat translucent consistency. Because it is slightly sweet, rice milk works well as a vegan milk substitute in vegan dessert and soup recipes.

Sunlight, vitamin D and bone health

To help prevent osteoporosis, a suitable plant-based diet as well as different fruits, nuts and vegetables will help along with plenty of sunshine.

Unlike other essential vitamins, which must be obtained from food, vitamin D can be synthesized in the skin through a photosynthetic reaction triggered by exposure to UVB radiation. The efficiency of production depends on the number of UVB photons that penetrate the skin, a process that can be restricted by clothing, excess body fat, sunscreen, and the skin pigment melanin.[81]

Without sufficient vitamin D, bones can become thin and brittle. A lack of vitamin D can also lead to rickets in children and osteomalacia, or soft bones, in adults.

Vitamin D helps the modulation of cell growth in the body as well as the neuromuscular and immune function and the reduction of inflammation.[82]

Michael Holick, a medical professor and director of the Bone Health Care Clinic at Boston University Medical Center, says: "The primary physiologic function of vitamin D is to maintain serum calcium and phosphorous levels within the normal physiologic range to support most metabolic functions, neuromuscular transmission, and bone mineralization."

Most people meet at least some of their vitamin D needs through exposure to sunlight. Solar ultraviolet (UV) B radiation with a wavelength of 290–320 nanometers penetrates uncovered skin and converts cutaneous 7-dehydrocholesterol to previtamin D3, which in turn becomes vitamin D3. Season, time of day, length of day, cloud cover, smog, skin melanin content, and sunscreen are among the factors that affect UV radiation exposure and vitamin D synthesis.

UVB radiation does not penetrate glass, so exposure to sunshine indoors through a window does not produce vitamin D.[83]

Any excess vitamin D3 that is produced during exposure to sunlight can be stored in our body fat and used during the winter, when less vitamin D3 is produced in our bodies.

Although the sun is closest to the earth in the winter, the sun's rays are entering at a more oblique angle (zenith angle) and more UVB photons are efficiently absorbed by the ozone layer, because the more oblique angle causes the UVB photons to pass through the ozone for a greater distance. In addition, with the more oblique angle there are fewer photons per unit area striking the earth. Time of day, season, and latitude all influence the zenith angle of the sun.

However, below 37° and closer to the equator, more vitamin D3 synthesis occurs in the skin throughout the year. Similarly, in the early morning or late afternoon, the zenith angle is so oblique that very little if any vitamin D3 is produced in the skin even in the summer.[84]

Concerns about skin cancer

Michael F. Holick talks about the dangers of too much sun in his article "Sunlight and vitamin D for bone health and prevention of autoimmune diseases, cancers, and cardiovascular disease." He says: "There is great concern about any exposure to sunlight causing skin damage, including skin cancer and wrinkling. Chronic excessive exposure to sunlight and sunburn incidents during childhood and young adult life significantly increase the risk of nonmelanoma basal and squamous cell carcinomas.

The most serious form of skin cancer is melanoma. It should be recognized that most melanomas occur on non sun-exposed areas and that having more sunburn experiences, having more moles, and having red hair increase the risk of the deadly disease.

Chronic excessive sun exposure also damages the elastic structure of the skin, increasing the risk of wrinkling. However, on the basis of our understanding of the efficiency of sun exposure for producing vitamin D_3 in the skin, it is reasonable to allow some sun exposure without sun protection, for production of adequate amounts of vitamin D_3."

The best time to sunbathe is when the dangers of ultraviolet rays are at a minimum, for example before 10am or after 3pm. This can vary by season and also by geographical area. Ten to 20 minutes of sun each day during these times can be healthy.

If your diet includes a plentiful amount of fruits and vegetables, which have many anti-cancer and antioxidant ingredients, the negative effects of ultraviolet and other harmful rays on the body will be greatly reduced. These antioxidants protect the body against free radicals. By eating a lot of meat and dairy you're not providing your body with any antioxidants but instead many carcinogens which weaken our body so we find it hard to fight free radicals and other carcinogens.

Other sun-dependent pathways[85]

There are many health benefits we gain from the sun. Here are just a few:

Direct immune suppression: Exposure to both UVA and UVB radiation can have direct immunosuppressive effects through the unregulation of cytokines (TNF-α and IL-10) and increased activity of T regulatory cells that remove self-reactive T cells. These mechanisms may help prevent autoimmune diseases.

Alpha melanocyte-stimulating hormone (α-MSH): Upon exposure to sunshine, melanocytes and keratinocytes in the skin release α-MSH, which has been implicated in immunologic tolerance and suppression of contact hypersensitivity. α-MSH also helps limit oxidative DNA damage resulting from UVR and increases gene repair, thus reducing melanoma risk, as reported 15 May 2005 in Cancer Research.

Calcitonin gene-related peptide (CGRP): Released in response to both UVA and UVB exposure, this potent neuropeptide modulates a number of cytokines and is linked with impaired induction of immunity and the development of immunologic tolerance. According to a report in the September 2007 issue of Photochemistry and Photobiology, mast cells (which mediate hypersensitivity reactions) play a critical role in CGRP-mediated immune suppression. This could help explain sunlight's efficacy in treating skin disorders such as psoriasis.

Neuropeptide substance P: Along with CGRP, this neuropeptide is released from sensory nerve fibers in the skin following UVR exposure. This results in increased lymphocyte proliferation and chemotaxis (chemically mediated movement) but may also produce local immune suppression.

Endorphins: UVR increases blood levels of natural opiates called endorphins. Melanocytes in human skin express a fully functioning endorphin receptor system, according to the June 2003 Journal of Investigative Dermatology, and a study published 24 November 2005 in Molecular and Cellular Endocrinology suggests that the cutaneous pigmentary system is an important stress-response element of the skin.

How Sunshine Affects the Brain

Sunshine affects the brain via the interaction of the chemicals melatonin and serotonin, as well as vitamin D. When sunlight hits your eyes, your optic nerve sends a message to the gland in the brain that produces melatonin (a hormone that helps you sleep); the gland decreases its secretions of melatonin until the sun goes down again.

The opposite happens with the chemical serotonin; when you're exposed to sun, your brain increases serotonin (a hormone connected with feelings of happiness and wakefulness) production. When the ultraviolet rays from sunshine hit your skin, your body produces vitamin D, which helps you maintain serotonin levels. Generally, we're asleep or feeling lethargic during the dark hours, and physically and emotionally up during the day. This is the human circadian rhythm. We are able to function against these biological rhythms when we must (as night-shift workers do), but it can be hard on our bodies and minds. When we go without sunshine, some get seasonal affective disorder (SAD); people who suffer from this disorder get depressed during the times when there's not much sun, although they're typically fine in the warmer, sunnier months of the year. SAD is most prevalent in places where there are scant sunlit hours in the winter (such as Alaska) or where it's overcast for extended periods (in parts of north west America). SAD can often be treated with phototherapy that exposes the patient to full-spectrum light, which may be sunlight or artificial light. Being out in the sun isn't enough by itself as we need to soak up the sun's rays.

Avoid Sunscreen as much as possible

From an early age many of us have been conditioned to put on sunscreen whenever we go outside, and there are downsides to the use of sun-blocking chemicals.[86]

In his article: '*Your sunscreen might be poisoning you*' Dr. Arthur W. Perry said chemical sunscreens don't sit on your skin but soak into and: "quickly find their way into the bloodstream".

He added: "They scatter all over the body without being detoxified by the liver and can be detected in blood, urine and breast milk for up to two days after a single application. That would be just fine if they were uniformly safe but they're not."[87]

Do not be afraid of nature

Nature may not be perfect but still the natural system is in harmony with its surroundings. Every creature has its own role to play.

Although occasionally we see diseases in the wild, they are rare and do not come close to the sickness that occurs amongst humans.

Nature is our mother and our friend, not our enemy. So if we return to a natural lifestyle, we have nothing to lose except the stresses and sickness that go hand in hand with our modern day lives.

In 2012 I attended a meeting about veganism in Iran. I listened to a speech from Dr. Shoja Farrokhi, a vegan doctor who spoke about the nutrients that nature provides for animals living in the wild. He said in nature every animal eats a limited variety of foods yet obtains all of its nutritional needs. For example, elephants and giraffes mostly eat leaves yet don't suffer any deficiencies. He then asked why most of us think that nature has forgotten to provide a complete food for humans? And why do people think fruits and vegetables aren't complete foods or that they don't supply all our needs so that we have to drink the milk of another animal for our calcium supply? Other animals do not do this so why should we? He added that we mustn't be afraid as raw veganism was a natural and healthy diet for humans.

Fortunately we humans have access to a variety of delicious fruits, nuts and vegetables. Also as we can cultivate what we need we will always have access to a variety of nutritional foods thus reducing the risk of nutrient deficiencies.

If our civilization became more nature-friendly, it would greatly benefit us and we would get much better results in life. Organic agriculture and green energy are two smart ways to continue our civilization while remaining healthy.

Essential fatty acids in a natural diet

Omega-3 fatty acids (also known as n-3 fatty acids) are polyunsaturated fatty acids that are essential nutrients for health. We need omega-3 fatty acids for numerous normal body functions, such as controlling blood clotting and building cell membranes in the brain. Since our bodies cannot make omega-3 fats, we must get them through food. Omega-3 fatty acids are also associated with many health benefits, including protection against heart disease and possibly strokes. New studies are identifying potential benefits for a wide range of conditions including cancer, inflammatory bowel disease, and other autoimmune diseases such as lupus and rheumatoid arthritis.

Omega-6 fatty acids (also known as n-6 fatty acids) are also polyunsaturated fatty acids that are essential nutrients, meaning that our bodies cannot make them and we must obtain them from food. They are abundant in the western diet; common sources include safflower, corn, cottonseed, and soybean oils.[88]

Essential fatty acids can also be found in some plant sources like walnut, flaxseed, seed of linen and some kinds of seaweed[89], as well as in some green vegetables, such as Brussels sprouts, kale, spinach, and salad greens.

These plant food sources are healthy and usually don't make human blood acidic causing other health problems unlike the negative effect that fish can have on the human body.

Fish is a sea animal so putrefies in the air very quickly, more quickly than meat. This putrefaction creates poisons which we consume when we eat fish posing a risk to our system. This is also the case when it comes to fish oil. Like other animal products, fish is not necessary for our bodies, whether for its omega 3 or anything else.

Another important issue which should be considered is the ratio between omega 3 and omega 6 that we consume.[90]

A healthy diet contains a balance of omega-3 and omega-6 fatty acids. Omega-3 fatty acids help reduce inflammation, and some omega-6 fatty acids tend to promote inflammation. In fact, some studies suggest that elevated intakes of omega-6 fatty acids may play a role in Complex Regional Pain Syndrome, a condition where someone experiences constant severe pain. The typical American diet tends to contain 14 - 25 times more omega-6 fatty acids than omega-3 fatty acids.[91]

Raw vegans don't usually need most of the supplements out there, because a natural diet is rich in almost all the nutrients we need.

Why we have deficiencies in our body

As Frederic Patenaude explains the topic of deficiencies very well in his book "**The Raw Secrets**," he also includes a wise quote from Albert Mosséri in Chapter 10: Supplements and Super-foods on what causes deficiencies. He writes:

"If you are suffering from a deficiency, it may be caused by impaired assimilation, not by
a lack of nutrients in foods. Mosséri explains: Let's take the case of anemia which is an iron deficiency in a patient. The analysis shows it, but when we scrutinize the patient's diet, we do not find a lack of iron in most cases! Typically, there is plenty of iron in the diet. In fact, in pernicious anemia, there is an excess of iron-based pigments in all the internal organs. Hunter discovered that even in fatal cases, a great quantity of iron leached from the blood and was found in the spleen. This shows that there is more iron than is needed in the bodies of anemic people; it's just not being used.
Another proof that anemia is not caused by a lack of iron in the diet is that this disease regresses during fasting, when no food is eaten and no iron is provided for the body through the diet. During a short fast, we notice a marked increase in the red blood cell count. This shows that there are iron reserves in the body but for some reason they are not used. This proves that iron found in foods and iron accumulated in the tissues has not been appropriated, because assimilation is failing. This is called a faulty metabolism.
So we are not witnessing an iron deficiency in the diet, but a lack of iron absorption. This deficiency is not of an immediate dietary origin, but could be after a long time.
After a seven-day fast, the red blood cell count increases noticeably. But if the fast is longer, we will surely witness a reduction of red blood cells and other elements since the reserves will be depleted at some point. For this reason, no analysis should be done for several months after breaking a fast.

What do we gain by feeding anemic people iron-rich foods, when they already possess abundant iron reserves in their tissues, unused because they cannot be assimilated?
Albert Mosséri

Mangez Nature Santé Nature

Nearly everyone drinks milk as a calcium supplement, yet many end up suffering from osteoporosis anyway. No matter how much calcium they take, they will not get better until they discard the various causes that prevent calcium absorption or leach calcium from the body. These include: caffeine, excessive quantities of protein in the diet, cigarette smoking, inadequate vitamin D, salt intake (including sea salt) and certain medications.
I do not recommend routine supplementation. I believe supplements can also cause problems instead of solving them. I recommend instead eating a nutritious diet that provides you with all the vitamins and minerals that you need."

Vitamin B12; what we should know

Vitamin B12 was first isolated in 1948. It is derived exclusively from bacteria. Since that time, research has established that vitamin B12 is required for a number of important functions, including the synthesis of thymidylate, a substance necessary for DNA synthesis.

One of the biggest problems and biggest concerns that people have with their diet is deficiencies of certain nutrients like calcium, potassium, vitamin B12 and so on.

The easiest solution, which people turn to, is supplements, but this is still not the answer as many people's health does not improve after using supplements even over a long period. This is because like other health issues; we should know and treat the root of the deficiency, not the symptoms.

The "lack of protein" in vegetarian diets was a myth for decades. Now we know it is only a hoax, because it has been proven scientifically that no vegetarian suffers from a lack of protein (except those individuals who have a metabolic disorder and are unable to absorb protein).Vegetarians are generally healthier and stronger than omnivores.

Nowadays people don't worry about a lack of protein in vegetarian diets, but some people are concerned about a lack of B12.

In fact, there are too many principles concerning nature and the human body which have not yet been discovered. For example, it's possible that many micronutrients haven't yet been discovered. Also the discovery of vitamins and micronutrients are described as theories, not as facts, because these materials can't be seen yet under a microscope or any other tool. Of course it doesn't mean that it is false, because a theory is based on many experiments and results. For example an atom and a molecule are also theories as they cannot be seen, but all related industries like nuclear power and chemical materials are based on this theory.

A theory is never complete, so it's natural that sometimes we see different results than what that theory concludes. So we should not rely on the theories, but instead, we should consider all experiences and all information then find the truth amongst the data.

On the subject of vitamin B12 there is still a lot to learn. But nevertheless, we can find interesting clues about B12 which has provoked much thought and debate.

Plants and animals can't produce vitamin B12. In nature, this vitamin can only be produced by some kinds of useful bacteria which live in soil and also in our digestive system. Some pesticides and chemicals kill these bacteria and sterilize the soil so can cause a deficiency of these bacteria in our foods. B12 is an amazing vitamin and its deficiency in the body can be very dangerous and can occur in some people regardless of their diet, whether vegans or meat eaters.

Symptoms of B12 deficiency can include numbness of the hands and feet, unsteadiness and poor muscular coordination, and even cognitive deficiencies such as confusion, mental slowness and memory problems. As declared in scientific references, B12 protects the nervous system and without it, permanent damage can result such as blindness, deafness, and dementia. Fatigue and tingling in the hands or feet, can be early signs of B12 deficiency.

Vitamin B12 is made by natural bacterial flora in the intestines. Organic plants may contain this useful bacteria (which is destroyed by the spraying of chemicals and anything which disarranges the flora bacteria balance in the human body) so organic foods can be a better source here as they are not affected by chemical poisons.

Avoiding unhealthy habits such as smoking, which can cause an imbalance in the body, is advisable to help prevent a vitamin B12 deficiency.[92]

According to vegans and vegan doctors from the Physicians Committee for Responsible Medicine (PCRM), vitamin B12 deficiency may occur among vegetarians, vegans and raw vegans, but not in all vegetarians. However most of them recommended that vegans should use B12 supplements regularly.

Dr. Zarin Azar, a gastroenterologist and a member of PCRM[93] advised several times on her Persian website and in her videos that every vegan should be careful about preventing/treating his B12 deficiency and take B12 sublingual supplements if needed. However, on the basis of her experiences during 20 plus years of working in the medical field, most of the vegans she met didn't have a B12 deficiency. She also recommends using the B12 supplement methylcobalamin because it's absorbed better than cyanocobalamin, but it's still controversial and opinions differ over this subject.

The reason why vitamin B12 deficiency is rare is because the human body has highly efficient mechanism to absorb and recycle this vitamin (however the statistics on this issue is also controversial). And the small intestine does a marvelous job of recycling B12, reabsorbing it from bile made by the liver.

Unfortunately chemical poisons, different herbicides and crop sprays are the main causes of killing useful bacteria which are the main producers of vitamin B12 by their fermentation.

Vitamin B12 deficiency doesn't just affect some vegans and vegetarians, even meat eaters and those who consume animal products can also get this deficiency. This is common as meat eaters' age as the absorption of B12 from meat may become much more difficult. An article on Tufts University's website explains:

"B12 in meat can be more difficult to absorb as you age because the vitamin is bound to protein in the meat and requires acid to break down. With age, your body produces less acid in the stomach."[94]

So all the propaganda which deny the dangers of meat eating for the human body and instead say we should consume meat or animal products to get our supply of vitamin B12, are not reasonable, because if this was true, so why do some meat eaters have a lack of B12, too? Eating animal products for the sake of vitamin B12 is not safe and wise, especially for older people and those people who suffer from digestive disorders and have a problem absorbing vitamins.

Other sources of Vitamin B12 such as meat, eggs and dairy are not always reliable because they have often been processed at high temperatures.

Protecting your intestinal flora

As the natural intestinal flora is very important to balance the body and produce useful nutrients like vitamin B12, so it's vital to keep it in balance. Frederic Patenaude described in his book "**Raw Secrets**" that what caused an imbalance in intestinal flora was the following:
"Normally, vitamin B12 is made in the intestinal flora with the help of beneficial bacteria.

So the most important thing is to make sure you do not destroy your intestinal flora with the following (in order of importance.)

1) The use of antibiotics

2) Many prescription drugs

3) Many popular herbal remedies that contain caffeine and multiple toxic substances.

4) Herbal intestinal cleanses

5) Repeated colonics

6) Overeating, which causes food to ferment and produce an array of poisons and acids that will impair the intestinal flora.

7) Regular consumption of frozen food

8) Coffee, tea and other stimulants

9) An excess of acidic fruits"

If you believe that you may have partly destroyed your intestinal flora (the use of antibiotics is often the main culprit), you may have a reason to worry about a vitamin B12 deficiency. In his article: '**Vitamin B12 Recommendations for Total-Vegetarians,**' Dr. Alan Goldhamer comments:

"Upon reflection, we should note that in a more primitive setting, human beings almost certainly would have obtained an abundance of vitamin B12 from the bacterial "contamination" of unwashed fresh fruits and vegetables, regardless of their intake of animal products. Human vitamin B12 deficiency is very unlikely to occur in such a setting. Only very small amounts of dietary vitamin B12 are needed because our bodies do a fabulous job of recycling this essential nutrient. A person living in the ancestral environment would have regularly consumed fresh fruits and vegetables that were not consistently, fastidiously cleaned, as we routinely do today. Our current unusual degree of hygiene is useful for combating many health threats — but may leave long-term, strict vegans vulnerable to the potential problem of vitamin B12 deficiency."

Although most people associate vitamin B12 deficiency with vegan diets, the majority of cases occur among people who regularly consume animal products. I have heard the same thing from several doctors and naturopaths who have had experience with B12-deficient individuals. They are mostly meat eaters. It proves that a lack of B12 in the diet is not the main cause of this deficiency, since animal products contain this vitamin. A lack of absorption, coupled with damaged intestinal flora, is the culprit."

Frederic Patenaude says:
"The most important things to do to avoid B12 deficiency; in order of importance are:
1) Avoid everything that destroys intestinal flora.
2) Include a sub-lingual, B12 supplement."
Consuming incompatible foods together at one time can also cause digestive problems, prevent the sufficient absorption of nutrients and also damage intestinal flora. Eating too much dried foods, which usually contain microscopic fungi, should be avoided along with salt, pickles and herbs which can affect intestinal flora as can onion, garlic, pepper and most bitter herbs.
Fasting and regular body cleansing can be helpful to increase the absorption of essential nutrients.
Many experts say that our liver stores as much vitamin B12 as our body needs for several years. On the basis of other evidence, the main problem in B12 deficiency is digestive disorders and also the body's inability to absorb nutrients[95].

As all vitamins, minerals and hormones work together in our body, any problems may be other deficiencies in our body. So we should treat and balance our body with natural methods.

As an example, and to understand it better, scientists have told us that a lack of vitamin C can cause gum disease, osteoporosis and many other diseases. It is true, but if a person eats meat and junk food all the day which doesn't contain vitamin C, and at the same time consumes 1000 mg. vitamin C pills to compensate then this would not mean that he or she was healthy. This is because the problem is not only a lack of vitamin C but usually it is accompanied by a lack of calcium and other problems. Also while the body is acidic and out of balance, it increases the risk of catching other diseases and the first step in a correct treatment is to alkalize the body and so return it to its normal and natural pH.

Vitamins are very sensitive to environmental situations such as temperature while overusing them is harmful and wastes the body's energy to collect and repulse extra poisonous matters. So vitamin pills are not a good solution over a long period.

On the topic of supplements in general, Dr. Douglas Graham argues in his book Nutrition and Athletic Performance that supplementation has proven to be an inadequate and incomplete method of supplying nutrients as scientists cannot match nature's refined balances. He says that since an estimated ninety percent of all nutrients are as yet undiscovered, why would we want to start adding nutrients to our diet one at a time rather than eating foods whole? Most nutrients are known to interact symbiotically with at least eight other nutrients and considering this, the odds of healthfully supplying any nutrients in its necessary component package becomes "infinitesimally minute". More to the point he adds: "there has never been a successful attempt to keep an animal or human healthy, or even alive, on a diet composed strictly of nutritional supplements".

Another side to the equation is that low serum B12 levels do not necessarily equate to a B12 deficiency. Just because there is a low level of B12 in the bloodstream, this does not mean there is a deficiency in the body as a whole, it may well be utilized by the living cells (such as the central nervous system). More reliable tests appear to be that of homocysteine levels and Methyl Malonic Acid tests[96].

Looking at all the information on deficiencies I would still prefer to take some supplements in an emergency situation. If I did develop a B12 deficiency I would not eat meat and unhealthy foods to solve a health problem as I would be adding several other risks and damages.

The positive effects of raw veganism is still worthwhile and fortunately B12 supplements do not have too many side effects over time because it is a water soluble vitamin so it's easier for the body to repulse through the kidneys if we eat more than we need. But we neither need nor should overuse anything.

And while meat eating cause many diseases that forced people to use tons of poisonous medical drugs to alleviate the pain. So that veganism/raw veganism is still worth it if we have to take only one kind of supplement (B12).

In total, we have to endeavor to live in a manner that is compatible with nature consuming organic foods as much as possible.

A Natural Life

Most people think the average age a person lives to is 70 to 80 years. From a natural health point of view I do not believe this to be true.

Real and true health means a long and happy life. No one really dreams of a life full of disease and misery. True health means no disease. All diseases have a cause which can be discovered and treated.

If we take the example of decay in our teeth; animals that had lived in the wild and followed a natural vegan diet have no corrosion in their teeth. While in humans teeth, which are the last organs of body to develop, often wear out quickly. However, it is a debatable subject because no one has really checked the dental health of all animals in the wild.

According to WHO decaying teeth is a localized, post-eruptive pathologic external process, involving hard tooth tissue and the formation of cavities. There is demineralization of teeth by acids produced in the oral environment, due to action of oral acidogenic bacteria on carbohydrates found in cooked food and drinks. Animals are either herbivorous or carnivorous or both, and survive on uncooked, raw food, rich in fiber, which needs a lot of chewing to digest, thereby cleansing the teeth naturally. It is like brushing teeth and massaging gums the natural way. But tooth decay is common in pets like dogs, which are often fed cooked food and junk food like biscuits[97].

All denatured foods rob the body of minerals. The excess acid in foods robs the body of calcium and other bases.

Any factor, physical, nutritional, emotional, etc., that perverts or impairs nutrition will cause the teeth to decay. Poor health, impaired nutrition, perverted metabolism, however produced, affect all the structures and functions of the body in varying degrees and any effort to preserve or restore integrity that ignores the cause of general impairment must fail.

Soft diets, which require no work of the teeth and jaws in chewing, aid in producing dental decay. No tooth can have adequate nutrition unless it is used. Easting soft mushy food does not give the teeth proper exercise. Raw foods are best. A tough, fibrous diet not only gives the teeth and jaws much needed exercise, but also cleans the teeth. The conventional, unnatural and highly refined, cooked diet leaves the mouth and teeth dirty.[98]

It is the following important factors which contribute to tooth decay[99]:

Poor food quality: Optimal health is dependent on optimal nutrition which comes from optimal foods. So, the first step is to avoid all processed and packaged foods. They are of low quality and have very little nutrition. While some packaged and processed foods might be fortified, these vitamins are synthetic and are barely absorbed by the body.

Poor food absorption: Many people on Western diets or SAD (Standard American Diet) cannot properly absorb the nutrients they eat because their guts have been damaged from years of poor quality, processed and denatured foods.

Teeth, like bones, are living organs. While they renew themselves much slower than softer organs, like your skin or your liver, teeth are constantly breaking down and replacing their cells. In a healthy person, new dentin and enamel is constantly being generated from vitamins, minerals and enzymes in your bloodstream and pushed out through microscopic tubules to the outer layers of your teeth. With enough vitamins and minerals in the right ratios, teeth will constantly remineralize and regenerate themselves naturally, and do not need treatments such as fluoride to remain healthy.

Animals which are kept by humans often suffer tooth cavities because they are forced to live and function outside of their natural environment. For example, cows in animal farming which are often forced to work harder, produce more milk than they naturally would and are fed in a small area with food that is less nutritious such as dried grass instead of fresh grass. When animals are completely free they are not under stress so they have more rest, produce milk only for their babies (less than the amount which humans squeeze out of them) and feed on different herbs in different areas with different soils. But now it is even worse because in some animal factories, cattle are fed with soy or corn or even the corpse of other animals which is turned into powder.

Natural foods such as fruit and vegetables means natural for the digestive system and the whole body. So the natural food which is compatible with our body system doesn't need to be cooked. Animals don't have a stove or a microwave in nature, but humans burn their food with these artificial instruments and then believe they have eaten natural food.

The natural pH of the human body

According to studies[100] a healthy body is slightly alkaline at about pH 7.4. Everything which causes acidity in the body along with too much alkaline, is poisonous for the body and should be avoided. All animal foods such as meat, dairy and eggs make the human blood acidic, as well as most cooked foods. So they cannot be our natural food and this is why they cause many diseases.

Natural food for humans should taste good in their original state such as fruits, vegetables, nuts and some seeds. These foods help the human blood to remain a little alkaline, as its natural state should be.

We are really not supposed to get sick as we age but instead to pass different stages of life, like any other creature on Earth passes all the stages from birth to death. So to become weak in our old age in comparison with youth is a different concept than becoming sick. The first is a natural phenomenon while the second is not.

Diseases are good signs which inform us about our mistakes, whether we are aware of them or not. A wise person will always search for the roots of any problem to understand what is really happening.

Poisons and detoxification explained

Poison or toxins are two words which I use in this book repeatedly.
Most people think that only cigarettes, drugs, chemicals and polluted air are poisons, but in fact it covers a much broader area.
Materials that can be poisonous for the body are divided into the following three categories:
#1. Those foods and materials which are pure toxins for the body and have no health benefit like smoke and all fried foods.
#2. Those foods which may have some benefits for the body in small quantities but are addictive and so controlling the quantity we consume is hard such as hot peppers.
#3. Those foods which are beneficial for the body but if we overindulge, the excess amounts will become harmful. So natural foods and even pure water could be harmful in excess.[101]
Each plant also has natural poisons within, but the amount in ripe fruits is less than all other herbs while these little amounts of poisons in some ripe fruits are not harmful for the body, for example the resin-like substance which comes out of figs and protects the fruit from hungry insects; this is not harmful for us because the body has adjusted to fruits during evolution.[102] On the other hand, if too many poisons enter the body this can lead to sickness. A little toxin can be useful and even essential for the body to make it able to deal with all poisons.[103] As fruits contain the fewest possible toxins by their nature, so they are safe to use, much safer than poisonous cooked foods which can damage DNA[104], lead to cancer[105], and speed up the aging process.
Some poisons are very dangerous like pesticides and some appear in cooked foods such as acrylamide found in cooked carbohydrates which are more dangerous than natural poisons, so we should avoid them completely.
The human body doesn't need unhealthy foods at all and even low amounts of them are harmful for the body. So French fries, fried chicken or alcohol are pure toxins for the body.

Natural poisons in herbs should be avoided as much as possible such as foods with high amounts of natural toxins like tomatoes or beans. They do have some benefits for the body but they also have some toxins like Solanine in tomatoes especially in unripe tomatoes[106] or Lectin in beans[107].

Harmful herbs

There are some plants which are very poisonous for humans like toadstools (however mushrooms and fungus are diatoms, not herbs).

Also there are some herbs which won't immediately kill you but are harmful if used every day like tea and coffee. However these are issues for debate[108] Some of these herbs have some advantages, but they turn blood into an acidic state, repulse iron and prevent effective absorption of some foodstuffs especially when used daily.

In the case of soy some researchers claim that it can prevent the absorption of some vitamins (like vitamin B) and it is worse if that soy is changed by genetic engineering (GMO)[109], so it's better to avoid it or if we want to use it, use at most only once per week. There are also some cases where eating soy and soy products regularly can damage the thyroid[110]. It seems that Asian people are more resistant against the damages of soy, as they have been using soy for several decades but it is better to avoid soy as much as possible especially for western and non-Asian people.

Peanuts (which are part of the bean group) have dangerous microscopic fungus which can cause allergies and even death.[111] It should only be consumed in its fresh sprouted state, as long as you are not allergic and you want to enjoy it and do not consume it regularly.

Spices such as curry powder and black pepper are harmful for body as they taste bitter, hot or otherwise and unpleasant when eaten alone[112].

Also too much spicy food does not taste good to those who don't eat it regularly. For example, in Iran our national foods are moderate in spices so when we eat spicy Indian or Chinese food we feel bad.

I experienced this awful feeling when I went to Malaysia and visited a number of Chinese and Indian vegetarian restaurants there. In one case, I got gum sores for about three days. It was not joyful experience at all.

The toxicity rate among them is different. Some spices are toxic and dangerous like nutmeg, which is a powerful hallucinogen when eaten in sufficient quantities.

In natural nutrition, we don't need spices to make our food delicious because natural foods taste and smell good already.

If you don't want to stop using all spices, you can still eliminate the worst spices, especially hot peppers because they are toxic, as Frederic Patenaude wrote in his book '*Raw Secrets*':

"Hot peppers are especially toxic. They contain capsaicin, which is a very poisonous substance. You can easily prove to yourself the toxicity of hot peppers by observing your body's reactions after eating them. The mouth salivates, and the nose often runs with clear mucus or water. These are ways for the body to dilute the poison. The warm feeling that you get is the irritation of the digestive tract and stomach. The body temperature often rises as the body tries to get rid of this strong, toxic substance.

Another argument against hot peppers and spices is that children will refuse them. No one would give a hot pepper to a child. Pregnant and nursing women are advised to avoid them. Apparently, the taste of garlic and onions, and the spiciness of hot peppers can be tasted in milk the day after the mother eats them. I take this to be another proof that the body is rejecting the toxins found in these foods.

At first, when you stop using spices and salt, some foods may taste bland to you. That is because spices and salt greatly dull your senses and your ability to enjoy the flavor of natural foods. After a few weeks, you won't even miss spices anymore — and food will taste even better without them. The subtle, intense flavors of natural foods are imperceptible to the dulled palate of the condiment eater."

Tea, coffee and healthier alternatives

Tea and coffee are two of the most common unhealthy herbal drinks. Most nations didn't know them several centuries ago but now, they are very popular all over the world.

As mentioned thirty years ago in a Persian book which is written about natural hygiene[113] an experiment was carried out on two groups of dogs whereby one group was only fed water and another group was fed just tea and coffee. The first group of dogs which solely had water lost 15 grams of their body weight each day and finally died after 30 days, but the other group of dogs lost 30 grams of weight each day and died after 15 days. This experiment shows that tea and coffee are corrosive and disturb body detoxification.

The experiment was carried out on dogs, which of course differ to a human experience, but it is still clear that tea and coffee acidify the body. We should limit the consumption of such drinks and if possible, cut them out completely.

Personally, I felt better after I stopped drinking tea and coffee. My parents stopped drinking tea and it helped stop their stomach aches. But as they started drinking it again, their stomach aches returned. So they realized they should cut it out of their diet. (In Iran, coffee is not very popular).

We really don't need stimulant foods to feel better; we need to support our body with natural foods, enough exercise and support our mind by good and positive thoughts to feel well.

But the question is: why should we drink tea or coffee every day? Why should we need them to feel better while they are not our complete foods?

Tea and coffee are addictive[114]. Even if we want to use and enjoy some herbal drinks, we should be aware of the consequences on our body.

If you still want to have herbal drinks and are looking for a coffee or tea substitute, I can recommend some natural drinks which I enjoy from time to time such as licorice, thyme, peppermint, rosemary and leaves of the blackberry tree (which can be useful for diabetes). It's better if we use different herbs instead of the same one every day.

I believe that a natural diet is not boring but is more diverse than many people's current wearisome diet. In fact, one of the reasons that led me to become vegan was the excellent diversity of vital foods. You can make powder from the mentioned herbs and let them soak in water for 12-24 hours, then use these raw herbal drinks instead of burning the sensitive herbs with boiling water.

What I need to wake me up in the morning

If you want to eat something that helps to wake you up in the morning, I suggest you eat an apple. It can be really more effective than coffee[115]. I didn't believe it when I heard it first, but I tried it and now I know it works. If you have any doubt, just try it. If it doesn't work there could be other factors making you feel sleepy such as Candida in the body which drain energy levels and everyone (even raw-eaters) can have this.

Food combination rules

When following a healthy diet we need to be aware of which foods are compatible. If we combine incompatible foods when eating our meals, it can lead to health issues such as digestive problems, bloating, headaches, and kidney problems.

When starting a raw vegan diet, if we still experience some pains or sickness after the first detoxification period, it is often because we are eating incompatible foods together. This is certain to happen if we have followed a raw vegan diet for some time.

As a simple but very important rule when deciding what to eat, remember: the simpler, the better.

Here I have listed the groups of foods which are compatible with each other and incompatible when combined with foods from other groups in large amounts:

#1. Foods which grow in the soil like carrots and potatoes.

#2. Fruits and vegetables which grow on bushes as well as melons and kiwis.

#3: Fatty seeds such as sesame and flaxseeds.

#4. Arboraceous sweet fruits, such as banana, apple and oranges.

#5. Arboraceous fatty fruits, such as avocado and durian.

#6. Nuts

#7. Fruits which are a little sour such as lemons, limes and sour cherries.

Each of the above mentioned groups are compatible with their mates and incompatible with herbs from other groups, however there are different opinions on this subject and it's better to refer to experts in natural hygiene for more information, especially if you suffer from severe digestive problems.

There are rules that need to be followed to ensure you feel good following a healthy diet:

#1. **Do not combine acid with starch** as the acidity can either prevent the digestion of starches in the mouth, or can make it much more difficult and sometimes painful. Examples of this combination include: mixing tomatoes with cooked potatoes, mixing tomatoes with bread, and eating bananas with oranges. Oranges are acidic and bananas contain starch, even when they are ripe. Bananas are better eaten with fruits that contain less acidity such as sweet apples or mangos.

Don't combine starch and protein because it can cause digestive problems. The protein enzyme protease is acidic, while the starch enzyme amylase is alkaline, so when we use high amounts of starch and protein together, such as eating beans with bread, these enzymes will neutralize each other so the food will remain longer in the stomach and start to rot producing harmful compounds like alcohol, which is very harmful for the body.

#2. **Don't combine sweet foods with fatty foods** because fats (including seeds, nuts and herbal oils) take a long time to digest while natural sweet fruits can be digested very quickly. When we combine the two, the sweet food will stay with the fatty food and remain in our stomach longer than it should. As it rots in our stomach, harmful compounds such as alcohol will be produced causing our stomach to bloat, which in turn will make us feel more tired and so crave more.

In this case, I have had bad experiences personally. When I became vegan, I would eat dates and nuts together because they tasted good. But I found the combination of date palm and walnuts made me feel tired.

Of course in natural foods, a little fat and sweetness are often found together, for example grapes which is a sweet fruit but has a little fat in its seeds as well as date palm which contains a little fat. These combinations are well balanced as a little natural fat helps the body to absorb some minerals and vitamins better. In natural fruits, a little amount of fat exists along with high amounts of natural sugar such glucose and fructose. A little natural sugar can also be found in some nuts, but all things are balanced in nature.

Still, if you want to mix sweets and fats, eating nuts with sweet fruits is okay as long as you limit the amount. However, the more time you eat sweet fruits separately to nuts, the better you will feel.

#3. Sweet fruits/sugar and starchy foods shouldn't be eaten together because   like fats, starch takes longer to digest, keeping the sweet food in your system longer causing it to putrefy in the stomach. The result of this is bloating and other digestive problems. No wonder so many people suffer from gas. Some examples include: bread with jam, cakes and pastries of all kinds and baked beans, which contain sugar.

So it is clear that all pastries, cakes and cookies are harmful for the body, due to the combination of starch and sugar. All of these artificial foods are imbalanced and it's necessary to avoid them as much as possible. If you do want a treat I would recommend raw vegan cakes, which are made without any animal products, of course only to eat occasionally and in low amounts.

#4. Do not combine dried fruits with acidic fresh fruits. Fresh fruits are preferred in a natural diet but if you still want to eat dried fruits, it's better to avoid combining them with fresh fruits. They especially don't mix well with most acid and sub-acid fruits (like oranges).

#5. Use fats in moderation and in low amounts. Fats (including nuts, seeds and oils) are condensed sources of energy. They're harder to digest especially when they're eaten with other foods. So however using natural and essential fats are necessary for our health, overusing them can cause problems such as fatigue, lack of concentration, excess weight, diabetes and skin problems.

It is recommended that fats in our diet make up less than 15% of our total calorie intake each day. So for example if we consume 2,000 calories per day, our fat intake should be no more than 300 calories.

Also many raw food experts recommend that we don't combine nuts/seeds and oils together, because oils are very dense fats so it's difficult to digest. Also they don't contain any fiber (cellulose) which is necessary to keep our digestion system efficient. Of course to say the exact amount of fat we should be consuming for anyone depends on many things. For example for a raw vegan who has recently started a detox, it is better to avoid fat during this period. Or through the winter when often our bodies need more fat to stay warm, then we can increase our intake slightly. My rule is that I pay attention to what my body tells me and trust my instincts.

For someone with diabetes or high cholesterol, it is recommended they consume 40-50 grams of nuts or seeds every day, less than two tablespoons of vegetable oil per day or even better, to avoid oils. It is better to get the fat and solvable minerals required from fatty fruits, nuts and seeds.

#6. Do not combine different types of fatty foods within one meal. Fatty foods are quite difficult to digest. When many different kinds of fats are present within a meal, digestion is considerably slower. Examples of this combination include: nuts with avocados, nuts with oil, coconut with avocado, coconut with other types of nuts, etc.
It is still okay to combine 2-3 fatty foods in small quantities, for example combining walnuts, sesame seeds and pistachios in small amounts. But just don't make it too complicated.

#7. Don't combine different condensed foods. Potatoes, wheat (and other starchy foods), seeds and nuts are condensed foods. Such foods need a long time to digest, so if combined could produce problems. It is generally better to have only one kind of these foods in each meal.
Starch and sprouts can be combined with high amounts of vegetables as long as the combination doesn't become too complicated.

#8. Don't combine incompatible fruits. It's better to eat fruits as a complete meal and also stick to one type of fruit per meal. If more than one fruit is desired in one meal, only combine fruits which are compatible. Do not combine acidic fruits and non-acidic fruits together.
Watermelon or melon is better eaten alone and bananas don't mix with acidic fruits like oranges or kiwis, because bananas are starchy.

#9. Fruits should not be eaten after cooked foods. This is because as mentioned before about the inappropriate food combinations, cooked foods need a long time to digest while fruits are very simple to digest. When incompatible foods mix together, the simpler food (especially fruits) will start to rot and produce toxic substances like alcohol, while many micro nutrients will be wasted as well. Therefore, fruits should be consumed at least one hour before any cooked foods are eaten.

Essential rules for preparing and eating foods

#1. Unfortunately the majority of recipes do not consider health and instead, the taste is their only priority.

Healthy gluten-free recipes which do not require salt and are low in fat are recommended (especially for raw vegans). If you find a complicated and unhealthy recipe, avoid it or change it to a simpler and healthier recipe.[116]

#2. Drinking water immediately after eating foods, even after watery fruits, is not recommended because water dilutes acids and enzymes in the stomach and can cause digestive problems, flatus, constipation, indigestion and so on.

#3. Food mastication is very important. If we don't chew foods very well, they will be difficult to digest and end up rotting in our bodies.

#4. It is possible that if we even consume a little cooked food as a raw vegan, we will return to previous bad habits, but I think this depends on the will of the person. But anyhow, if you ever want to have some cooked foods, at least choose the healthier ones. Avoiding fried foods is not as difficult as that!

I would need to write another book to cover all the details I'd like to in this chapter but I've highlighted the most important points and would recommend you read more health-related books and increase your knowledge.

After understanding the true and natural manner of eating, there is no excuse not to start. So we should empower our spirit to achieve our eating goals. Based on my experience I believe the best choice is to be a raw-foodist as much as possible, however it may not be easy for everyone to do this. At least we can try our best to be a raw vegan most of time.

The Benefits of Soaking Nuts and Seeds

Nuts and seeds are delicious natural foods. Tree nuts and seeds contain a high concentration of fat and protein provided by nature to ensure that an actively growing sprout will have all the nourishment it needs. They are dense food sources so are hard to digest. So to say in an average way, we should only consume at most about 50 or 60 grams per day.

These valuable food sources are usually easy to store and can be for about one year. Any longer than this and they start to rot and lose most of their nutritional value. They also lose some of their water and moisture during storage and microscopic fungi, which are harmful for body, can start to grow on their crust, especially on walnuts.

Just like any other raw foods, nuts and seeds contain enzymes inside them. However, till the germination conditions for nuts and seeds are met—like moist soil, or in our case a soaking process, the enzymes in most nuts and seeds stay dormant, held hostage by so-called enzyme inhibitors (another brilliant natural mechanism to ensure the proliferation of the species).

When the conditions are right for seeds to start growing, the enzymes within them break free from those inhibitors, and start breaking down nutrients into simpler chemical forms, thus making them easier for digestion and assimilation, lessening the burden on our digestive organs.

It's not possible to consume nuts and fatty seeds in high amounts like fruit, therefore storing them are unavoidable and so these enzyme inhibitors are very useful for this reason. If not, the seeds will rot very soon without these inhibitors.

But these enzyme inhibitors, which are clearly reduced in fresh nuts, are not useful for our bodies.

When we eat raw nuts and seeds, we also eat the enzyme inhibitors that prevent the seed from sprouting. This outer coating is a problem for us because it is made up of nutritional enzyme inhibitors and toxic substances. These enzymes inhibitors bind to our own enzymes and prevent them doing what they are meant to do. When it comes to our absorption of nutrients, it would cause different problems.

Consuming those tough little enzyme inhibitors puts a strain on our digestive system, since they will prevent our own enzymes from breaking down the food in our digestive tracts, inhibiting absorption of precious vitamins and minerals.

Luckily, Mother Nature evened the playing field by giving us humans the intelligence to find a way around this dilemma. Simply by soaking nuts and seeds in water, you release these toxic enzyme inhibitors and unlock the full vitality contained within the nuts and seeds. Also most of those microscopic fungi and their toxins will be released into the water, too, so that water isn't useful for us anymore. But it is still good to water flower or garden.

Soaked nuts are easier to digest, more absorbable and do not put excess pressure on the pancreas (which can cause it to enlarge).

Soaked nuts don't stick to our teeth so it helps our oral health, too. They're also better to use in raw salad dressings or other raw food recipes after softening.

Nuts taste better after soaking, particularly walnuts because soaking helps to remove the bitter taste.

Those nuts with a dark cortex, like walnuts and almonds, need soaking for at least 2-3 hours, while seeds need less soaking time (about 10-20 minutes). Soaking is beneficial at least to remove dust especially from those nuts which are not fresh[117].

Soaking and Sprouting Chart

Raw seeds, grains and nuts should be soaked before using to make them easier to digest.

After soaking, be sure to rinse seeds and nuts thoroughly with fresh pure water until it runs clear to remove the enzyme inhibitors that have been released into the water. It is also recommended to rinse some seeds and nuts (especially walnuts) two to three times during the soak.

After soaking, you can dehydrate at 105 degrees until the nuts/seeds are completely dry. Store them in the refrigerator or freezer to keep them fresh. Use within three days but the fresher, the better.

The following chart gives a guideline for soaking and sprouting times of the most common seeds, nuts and grains[118].

Seed, Nut or Grain	Soak Time	Sprout Time
Walnuts	4 hours	N/A
Almonds	8-12 hours	12 hours
Sesame Seeds	8 hours	1-2 days
Sunflower Seeds (hulled)	2 hours	2-3 days
Cashews	2-2 ½ hours	N/A
Pecans	4-6 hours	N/A
Pumpkin Seeds (hulled)	8 hours	1 day
Flax	8 hours	N/A
Nuts (all others)	6 hours	N/A
Green Peas	12 hours	2-3 days
Lentils	8 hours	12 hours
Millet	8 hours	2-3 days
Mustard	8 hours	2-7 days
Oat Groats	6 hours	2 days
Fenugreek	8 hours	3-5 days
Corn	12 hours	2-3 days
Rye	8 hours	3 days
Chickpeas	12 hours	12 hours
Clover	4-6 hours	4-5 days
Barley	6-8 hours	2 days
Wild rice	9 hours	3-5 days
Alfalfa	8 hours	2-5 days
Red Clover	8 hours	2-5 days

Grains: are they natural foods for us?

Some natural hygiene experts believe that grains and beans are not natural foods for us, because they contain large amounts of protein and starch and this feature makes them harder to digest. Most birds have a crop and gizzard, which help them to digest grains easily with the small stones they eat. Humans don't so therefore shouldn't eat grains.

Some grains, like wheat, contain too much gluten; a harmful protein which causes our bodies to produce mucus. Those that suffer with celiac disease, a digestive disorder that can damage the lining of the small intestine, have no way to ease their symptoms unless they avoid gluten.

Our bodies do not need grains and legumes, but if you want to consume them at least try to minimize the amount in your diet.

White bread and its damages on our health

There is no place for bread in a healthy diet, especially white bread, which I consider to be junk food. Raw breads are better alternatives, as is gluten-free bread.

The yeast in white bread affects the pH balance in our body making it acidic, as meat and dairy does, causing us to draw on our calcium reserves to alkalize body which then weakens our bones. This makes us more vulnerable to osteoporosis.

Acrylamide

Bread also contains the chemical compound Acrylamide, which has been found to increase the risk of several types of cancer when given to lab animals.

The American Cancer Society said Acrylamide has: "probably always been present in some foods, but this wasn't known until Swedish scientists first found it in certain foods in 2002."[119]

The chemical compound, also found in potato chips and French fries, is formed when bread is heated higher than 250° F (120 °C). Cooked starch such as rice and steamed potatoes are better because they are boiled in water.

Acrylamide can be 100 times more dangerous than other toxins in foods. This toxic chemical material can cause cancer, infections, impotence and damage to the nervous system.

For more information about the dangers of Acrylamide here are some credible references:

World Health Organization (WHO):
http://www.who.int/foodsafety/chem/chemicals/acrylamide/en

http://www.who.int/water_sanitation_health/dwq/chemicals/acrylamide/en/
http://www.who.int/mediacentre/news/notes/2005/np06/en/

Health Canada:

http://www.hc-sc.gc.ca/fn-an/securit/chem-chim/food-aliment/acrylamide/index-eng.php
http://www.hc-sc.gc.ca/fn-an/securit/chem-chim/food-aliment/acrylamide/major_pathway-voie_09_mar_05-eng.php
The QR codes of links above in sequence (from left):

http://www.hc-sc.gc.ca/fn-an/securit/chem-chim/food-aliment/acrylamide/acrylamide_level-acrylamide_niveau_table-eng.php

FDA:

http://www.fda.gov/Food/FoodSafety/FoodContaminantsAdulteration/ChemicalContaminants/Acrylamide/

European Union:

http://ec.europa.eu/food/food/chemicalsafety/contaminants/acrylamide_en.htm
The QR codes of links above in sequence at next page (from left):

New Scientist Magazine:
http://www.newscientist.com/article/dn2476-acrylamide-in-food-a-major-concern.html

National Biotech information:
http://www.ncbi.nlm.nih.gov/pubmed/15366289

Natural Health Way:
http://www.naturalhealthway.com/articles/acrylamide/acrylamide.html
The QR codes of links above in sequence in next page (from left):

Gluten

Gluten is the main structural protein found in all forms of wheat as well as some grains. This sticky protein has no nutritional benefit for our bodies and just puts extra pressure on our digestive system.

Gluten is composed of two types of similar proteins called gliadins and glutenins. Glutenins are simple proteins that can be easily broken down with secretions from the stomach, pancreas and small intestine. However, gliadins are bulkier and resistant to acidic secretions in the stomach. Enzymes further down in the digestive tract cannot chew them up, so they remain insoluble and stick to the small intestinal tube. Gliadins are formed from crossbreeding wheat plants and genetically modifying them for high production at harvest (i.e. altering wheat DNA to select genes that are resistant to harsh weather, fertilizer absorption and pesticide damage[120].

When gluten is cooked it produces mucus which provides a suitable environment for harmful bacteria, fungi and microbes to breed. This is the main cause of a common cold, because our body is forced to get rid of this harmful mucus[121].

Another condition that stimulates an immune response in the body to gluten exposure, yet does not cause intestinal damage is classified as a wheat allergy. It is less harmful than celiac disease because it involves the body responding to gluten as an allergic reaction, rather than an attack of healthy tissue by an autoimmune reaction. Allergic reactions are a buildup of a subpopulation of white blood cells to the skin or mucus area when a foreign allergen, or in this case gluten, comes into contact with it. These white blood cells are called basophiles and they secrete chemical messengers called histamines, which signal your body to produce defense mechanisms such as mucus, tears, pain and inflammation. These "protection strategies" are carried out because your body suspects that gluten is attacking it. Depending on the route of exposure to gluten, an allergic reaction to wheat can affect the skin, gastrointestinal tract or respiratory tract. Also, the intensity of the allergic reaction can vary with the type of gluten food product, for example eating cereal could produce a small rash and eating toast could result in hives[122].

Some people have a gluten intolerance (for example people with celiac disease) so they should follow a gluten-free diet which I would recommend as part of a healthy diet for everyone.

Making bread with other grains such as corn or oats could be far better, as wheat grains contain the most gluten.

The importance of drinking pure water

The water that we drink should be pure, just like the foods we consume. The best drinking water for humans should be from sources such as mountain springs which are low in (inorganic) minerals.

In raw vegan, especially fruit-based, diets, most of the body's water needs come from the raw fruits and vegetables we consume but we still need to drink water.

Some health experts say that distilled water is best because the inorganic dissolved minerals in water are not very useful for the body but not everyone agrees with this.

Unfortunately due to environmental pollution, water from some springs contains a lot of pollutants. The water that we get from our faucets has travelled through pipes contains many pollutants such as chlorine, fluoride and dangerous chemicals from any corrosion in the pipes.

Most raw vegans (including me) dislike the smell and taste of chlorine in pipeline water so it's always better to use a water purification machine or at least boil it in a non-aluminum pot before chilling it. Boiling doesn't eliminate all pollutants but it's better than doing nothing. Using distilled water can be useful at least over short periods, because it helps to accelerate body detoxification. Drinking distilled water during a detox program helps to cleanse your kidneys, bladder and bloodstream since it is a natural chelator.

The chlorine found in pipeline water is harmful even when you use it to wash because the chlorine gas evaporates when the water gets warmer harming not only our insides but our hair and skin.

The added chemical fluoride in water is very harmful for our brain and kidneys.[123] Many believe it's necessary to maintain healthy teeth but this is achieved with a healthy diet, good hygiene and enough vitamin D, which is necessary for the health of our bones and teeth. Most people have tooth decay even with fluoride in our water, so adding fluoride to drinking water is not the answer.[124]

The corrosion and fungi found in our drinking water pipes is often eliminated by adding chlorine to kill dangerous parasites and hazardous bacteria in the water. But I think using a water purification machine is the best solution at this time. We can only hope scientists come up with a better solution to this problem.

Salt: Myths and Realities

Common salt (NaCl or sodium chloride) is a mineral which provokes many different opinions, so it's necessary to find out more before we decide whether to remove it from our food.

But if, after reading this chapter, you still want to use salt I recommend you use natural salt like sea salt and should avoid chemically refined salt as it's refined in very high temperatures and some very harmful chemicals are added to it during the process.[125]

When anyone speaks about the harmful effects of salt or the benefits of a salt-free diet, some people express concern about a lack of iodine if they were to eliminate salt.

Cases where there is an iodine shortage in the body stems from consuming an unnatural diet comprising of unhealthy cooked foods. Inorganic iodine is one of the most poisonous substances for the body, so like all minerals it should be natural and organic to be beneficial for the body. A healthy diet will provide all the iodine our body needs.

Recommended Iodine Intake

Adolescents and adults need about 150 mcg of iodine a day. Pregnant and breastfeeding women may need about 220 mcg a day.

Iodine is an essential mineral, meaning the body is not able to make iodine on its own, and iodine must be absorbed via nutrition or emergency medical supplementation under the supervision of medical professionals.

Iodine Plant Sources

Most plant sources grown on iodine rich soils are good sources of dietary iodine.

Depending on the quality of the soil, on average, a serving of vegetables or fruit could have about 10 mcg of iodine, but sometimes this could go as high as 1000 mcg (1 mg) per serving.

If one simply eats a mono meal of 15 bananas, the daily iodine requirements of 150 mcg have been met.

Strawberries are a fruit considered to be a rich source of iodine and one cup of strawberries has 13 mcg of iodine. A cup of strawberries is only about 46 calories, so many servings can be consumed.

A head of raw romaine lettuce is equal to about six to seven 90 oz servings and may contain between 20 mcg to 60 mcg of iodine.

Other foods thought to be rich in iodine are pineapple, coconut, and some nuts and seeds such as black walnuts, and hazelnuts.

Although not optimum foods, some lentils and white potatoes are considered good sources of iodine. However, because they are high in oxalate acid, there may also be evidence that these foods could possibly interfere with thyroid function.[126]

We know that salt is not an herb or a live creature, so it's an inorganic matter and this is enough to signify that it cannot count as a useful substance for the body which thrives on natural nutrition.

Salt is a killer for many types of fauna and flora except for xerophytes, which are plants which have adapted to survive even with a limited supply of water, or in very salty marshy habitats.

For aquatic creatures, which have adjusted to salt over millions of years, if the level of salt in the rivers and seas increases more than they are used to, such as in times of drought or other environmental disasters, it would cause some types of creatures to die. If the level of salt in the sea or lake increases too much, there would be no animals living there, like The Dead Sea[127] in the Middle East.

The only exception are xerophilous animals; those that have adapted to very dry conditions, like some cows, goats and deer, which sometimes lick salt stone if they see it. It isn't entirely clear why these animals lick salt but it's important to note that just because salt is needed by some animals it doesn't follow that it's also needed by humans. The body of each animal is very different, especially if we compare two completely different species.

It's very clear that we humans are not interested in licking salt at all because it's intolerable for us and we cannot eat salt alone, so this should be a natural guide to whether we eat salt or not.

We know that sea water is lethal for plants and animals which live on land, so we cannot use salty sea water in agriculture. Drinking this saline water is very dangerous for humans too and can cause a multitude of physical and mental problems (like vomiting and hallucinations) and even death if too much is consumed.

So if we understand that salt isn't suitable for humans, why do many of us still consume this useless stuff every day?

In fact, the most dangerous factor in the perversion of our diet is salt. This is because most cooked foods are unsavory without salt, so for nearly as long as we have been cooking foods we have been using salt.

I believe there is a direct relation between using salt in cooked foods and our addiction to unhealthy and unnatural nutrition.

As salt is very addictive some people even add it to raw foods like salads. This is because their taste buds do not enjoy natural foods anymore.

Charlotte Gerson, the daughter of Max Gerson - one of the pioneers of a natural diet - didn't use salt at all and is now a very healthy 91-year-old. In an interview she did say she had once eaten salty foods at a party in a raw vegan restaurant in the USA and had felt an abnormal thirst and an inflamed feeling in her mouth, which were not pleasing, she said[128].

Salt (sodium chloride) has many negative effects on our body's biochemistry and causes many problems like hypertension, which can be fatal[129], and in turn damage vessels and the heart muscle[130], affects the kidneys[131], causes the body to reject calcium and can cause osteoporosis[132], inner hemorrhages[133], inner wounds, stomach cancer[134] and asthma[135].

The thirst we feel after eating salty foods is a sign that salt is poisonous and the body needs more water to flush it out to stop it killing our cells[136].

Salt upsets the balance of body and mind because of its dangerous negative effects on blood biochemistry. Salt also kills useful bacteria in the body, so this can cause many problems.

Natural fruits, vegetables, nuts and seeds supply our body with the sodium we need. Humans have been getting the sodium they need without having to add salt, simply by just consuming natural food, for millions of years.

The lack of sodium in the body isn't only caused by a lack of sodium in our foods, but also too much sodium excreted from the body, such as metabolic disorders or perspiring too much, which fortunately raw vegans don't suffer from.

Adding salt to our food is not a good way of treating a lack of sodium in the body, because first, it seems that salt can't hydrolyze in the body. This means that sodium and chlorine in salt cannot be useful for the body. (Please note that to hydrolyze is different from to dissolve in water. Salt should hydrolyze to be useful, which means separating sodium and chlorine ions).

There is too much controversy surrounding this subject. I have heard of cases where people, who were near death through excessive perspiring and thus repelling too much sodium, were healed by eating a little salt. However, we should not forget that as salt is very addictive and consuming excessive amounts is harmful. Of course people's resistance against the damages of salt differs, but still the salt addiction couldn't be counted as something useful.

If we suppose that salt hydrolyzes in the body, the sodium in it would not be useful for the body because the body needs organic minerals while salt is a dead material like soil. However I don't believe that salt is hydrolyzed because there is no enzyme in body to digest this dead material. In addition to this all minerals, vitamins and hormones work together, not alone.

If our body can't hydrolyze salt then the sodium it contains can't be useful for the body at all, as we can't eat calcium bicarbonate for its calcium, or iron corrosions for iron, or chemical fertilizer for its potassium. Because such materials cannot be useful for the body then they are very dangerous to consume. So eating salt to absorb its sodium or chlorine is pointless as our body cannot separate its ions.

Sodium and chlorine are two important elements for the body and natural foods contain enough amounts of them. But there is no dead salt (in the form of sodium chloride) in plants or even animals and this is another sign of the difference between organic and inorganic elements.

The sodium potassium balance is very important too. As we see in food value tables, the potassium of natural foods (especially fruits) is several times more than their sodium content, while salt just repels potassium from our bodies.

We drink water but not for its oxygen. So the reason why some mammals lick salt stone is something we don't know yet. But if we feed more salt to these animals, their liver would soon be damaged. Salt poisoning has been reported in virtually all species of animals all over the world.[137]

We need to rethink our consumption of salt.

Sodium deficiency is a separate subject from salt. It has different causes[138] and has some signs to diagnose[139]. But, like all other deficiencies in body, it is related to our nutrition. If the body becomes healthy and its biochemistry remains normal we absorb and get rid of sodium as we should.

Some soldiers based in hot places like the south of Iran, have experienced a crick in the neck due to the fact they are active in very hot conditions and sweat more. They also tend to eat a lot of poor nutritional food which are not natural. So there is a clear and direct relation between unhealthy foods and a lack of sodium along with other minerals.

Based on the experiences of some raw vegan and natural holistic experts, often consuming too many vegetables and vegetable juices with high oxalic acid like spinach and tomatoes can lead to a sodium shortage. So some people have to limit their use of vegetable juices if they are at risk. A natural fruit-based diet and using vegetables with less oxalic acid, is the best way to prevent a sodium shortage in the body.

Over time salt has a very bad effect on the brain and nervous system if consumed every day. In previous centuries, salt was consumed even more than today and people would cover almost all foods with salt to preserve them because they did not have a refrigerator. Granted they didn't have the stresses which people have these days, but still there were many cases of psychosis and mental diseases.

If you are used to a salty diet and always add extra salt to your foods, it may have some negative effects if you eliminate it suddenly from your diet. Salt has very bad effects on the body's biochemistry and is very addictive, so removing it is not always easy.

The best way to get free from salt addiction is reduce it gradually and don't add extra salt to your food (especially to salads and raw foods). Also you may be able to substitute salt with sodium-rich herbs in your foods, until you get accustomed to the change in your diet.

By removing salt, switching to a raw vegan diet is usually easier than eating salt-free cooked foods. But if you want to eat a little cooked food, salt-free recipes are the best option.

As we follow a natural diet more and more, there are fewer reasons to use salt and other seasonings.

I became accustomed to a low salt diet during my childhood, because my mother didn't like salty foods and didn't use too much salt in her cooking. Sometimes my mother forgot to add salt to our meals and I didn't even notice it at all. So I could remove salt easily from my diet and now I enjoy my raw vegan diet more than before.

A salt-free diet

To conquer salt cravings, there are different alternatives which make it so much easier to eliminate dead salt from our daily diet.

Frederic Patenaude has written some very interesting facts about salt and suggests a good alternative for salt in his book 'The Raw Secrets' chapter 15: Salt, Spices and Condiments:

"Salt kills life, which is why we preserve foods in salt. It is an antibiotic, which means "anti-life". If you put salt on a fresh cut in your skin, you will be able to feel its effects. It will burn you. Salt can accumulate in the body. It causes the body to retain water in order to dilute the salt in the tissues and prevent harming the cells. Excess salt is deposited at various places in the body such as on the artery wall. Blood flow is thereby disrupted and the result is high blood pressure.

Sea salt is not much better than other types of salt. Sea salt is just rock salt diluted by the ocean. The body has no use for it when it has access to the natural sodium contained in fruits and vegetables.

Before the Europeans arrived on this continent, native people did not use salt and were in excellent health. Many cultures throughout the world never used salt until the Europeans introduced this poison to them. After they started including salt into their diet, their health progressively deteriorated, although there were several other contributing factors to this deterioration.

Animals don't eat salt, unless they get tempted into licking a salt source which occurs naturally. Their instinct is better than ours, but not 100% perfect.

They can also make mistakes and be fooled by salt. Anyhow, salt licks are rare and most animals never come across such a source.

When you stop eating salt, it will take many months for your body to reject it. Some days you may taste salt in your mouth, although you may not have eaten it in weeks. It is more proof that the body is rejecting the salt and not using it. You may urinate more at night for a while, even many months, until the body has rejected all the salt. Complete "desalinization" of the body may take years.

To replace salt, I have come up with a natural seasoning using celery. Simply dehydrate slices of celery (in very large quantities) in a dehydrator or oven (at a low temperature.) When they are completely dried, turn them into a powder using a coffee grinder. This will make a nice, naturally salty seasoning that you can use to replace salt.

You can do the same with other vegetables to add additional flavor to this seasoning.

Dried purple cabbage powder is especially good in salads."

To add to this, during my research I became familiar with another substitute for salt which is an herb called salicornia, which grows in salty water and tastes salty (but stronger than celery). I don't have access to salicornia to try it yet, but it grows in Korea and also some European countries (in the areas near the sea) and can be used in salads, both fresh and in a powder form.

I have discussed with doctors eliminating dead salt completely from the diet, and they haven't always agreed with me but they did agree that salicornia is much better than dead sodium chloride[140]. It can also be useful especially for people addicted to salt or those individuals who lack sodium. Still, too much sodium (from any source) is harmful, so it's better to first ask your health care practitioner about the appropriate amount of this herb to use, depending on your health status.

Fruit: the great gift of nature

Fruits are very appealing to our palettes without having to do anything to them. This is in contrast to grains and most vegetables which need to be cooked to appeal to us.

As sweet fruits contain mono-saccharides (glucose and fructose), a major fuel for the human body, they should be a major part of a healthy diet.

Fatty fruits (nuts) contain necessary fats for the body as well as about 15-20% protein, so are very beneficial in small amounts.

Some additional facts about fruit, in brief:

Ripe fruits have the minimum amount of natural toxins, so they are beneficial for everybody.

Fruits, especially fruits from a tree, have the least risk of parasite pollution, making them the cleanest of foods.

Fruit trees provide nectar for bees and a habitat for birds and wildlife.

Fruit trees produce high amounts of oxygen which is beneficial both for humans and the environment.

Trees absorb more minerals from the soil so they need fewer fertilizers. Fruit trees also have more longevity than other herbs and can be used as compost after they die, so are very economical.

The aromatic compounds of fruits are beneficial for health while cause human to enjoy more:

Phenols are aromatic compounds that occur in essential oils of fruits. The benefits don't stop at the great fragrance though, because phenols have powerful antiseptic and antibacterial properties. These fragrant compounds can act as nerve stimulants and immune system stimulants.[141]

We should appreciate these gifts of nature and by planting and growing them using completely natural methods, we can enjoy their benefits for both our body and the environment.

However, we shouldn't fool ourselves and nature by using chemical fertilizers, pesticides and other poisons, which is harmful both for our bodies and the environment. Synthetic fertilizers tend to replenish only nitrogen, potassium, and phosphorus while depleting other nutrients and minerals that are naturally found in fertile soil.

Pesticides are used to kill the crop invaders. By eating food grown using pesticides we are ingesting these chemicals which reach the colon and remain there, making the colon toxic thus slowly poisoning the body.

Through countless studies, pesticides have been linked to Cancer, Alzheimer's disease, ADHD, and even birth defects. Pesticides also have the potential to harm the nervous system, the reproductive system, and the endocrine system. Pesticides can even harm fetuses because the chemicals can pass from the mother during pregnancy[142].

According to a study carried out by students from the University of Wisconsin, the combinations of commonly used agricultural chemicals, in concentrations that mirror levels found in groundwater, can significantly influence the immune and endocrine systems as well as our neurological health[143].

Organic agriculture and reducing chemical pesticides as much as possible is the solution, and this does not have a substitute in a completely healthy lifestyle.

So however difficult and in many situations, impossible to avoid non-organic fruits, at least we can reduce the pesticide residues in some way, such as washing them with 2% of salt water, which will remove most of the contact pesticide residues that normally appear on the surface of vegetables and fruits[144].

Breaking our bad eating habits

For those who have some knowledge about psychology know that habits, which are formed in our subconscious, have a very strong hold on our lives and affect the choices we make. To break bad habits can be difficult and a step by step approach should be taken.

As humans we usually imagine changing our habits will be too hard and so avoid trying to break them. For example all people know that cigarettes are poisonous and greatly damage our body, but millions of people smoke because they don't want to change.

When it comes to food, it becomes even harder for people to change their habits. In many cases, some people don't want to even consider it because they are used to eating traditional foods and they think changing their diet means limiting themselves. Some people even think if they don't eat traditional foods they will become sick.

It seems that almost all popular foods are declared "useful" or even "necessary" for the body. Even on the packaging of junk foods, such as potato chips, there is a table of ingredients which includes "energy" and "carbohydrates". There is no information about the harm and poisons of such foods, as they can often contain ingredients which are bad for our health, such as salt, or they are processed to a level where too many free radicals are produced, which are dangerous for the body.[145]

Many people love to hear good news about unhealthy foods. Sometimes they feel they need a reason to eat foods which they know are not good for them. For example when a doctor declares on TV there is no relation between saturated fats and heart disease, many people are glad of this news because it justifies their bad habits. If more people and more experts were talking about raw foodism and other healthy diets, more people would be ready to change their lifestyle for the better.

We should always remember that our brains are our most valuable asset in this material world. The most important function of the brain is to determine good from bad; without this happiness and well-being is impossible.

So, we should be independent thinkers. We shouldn't just accept what is dictated to us, even if it is said by "scientists", as no one is perfect.

We should be aware of our subconscious because it determines our destiny. We should always try to avoid all kinds of fanaticism which cause us to be ignorant of the truth so we never have to change our opinions and habits.

As an obvious nutritional fact, most traditional foods in many parts of the world are not healthy at all. For example, Iranian traditional foods are very fatty often involving too much bread and rice. Indian traditional foods are often spicy and intolerable for most people from other nations. Traditional foods are still better than fast food, but it's not a good reason to consider them perfect. The most crucial food for us is natural foods such as fruits.

If we want a healthy balanced life and a clean body which is strong enough to fight disease, then we should eat and live in a natural and healthy way.

Of course it's not always easy for everyone to resist food cravings. But different techniques to conquer food cravings such as some mind-control techniques will help kick bad eating habits.

When we have enough reasons to be happy and enjoy life then food is only a part of our enjoyment, not all of it. And then we will eat to live not live to only eat.

Contradictions in medical science

Scientific discoveries in the field of health and nutrition are made every day. As research is updated and new theories are formed we find there are many contradictions that can often be confusing. In his book *'Natural Cures "They" Don't Want You To Know About'* Kevin Trudeau talks about certain scientific "facts" that were later proven to be unreliable. Trudeau writes:

"The medical industry presents itself as the only source of truth when it comes to health, illness and disease. They use words like credible scientific evidence, scientifically tested, scientifically proven.

The fact is that what they are really presenting are theories, and these theories constantly change.

Here is an example of "medical facts" that have been proven to be wrong:

Bloodletting was once proven to cure most illnesses. Now it is considered totally ineffective.

Margarine was considered much healthier than butter. Now research suggests that the exact opposite is true.

Alcohol in all forms was said to be 100 percent unhealthy and therefore should not be consumed. Then the medical community said that red wine is actually healthy for the heart but not other forms of alcohol. Now "medical science" says that all alcohol in moderation actually has health benefits.

Chocolate and oily foods were touted to be a cause of acne. Now research suggests that they do not contribute in any way to acne.

Medical doctors touted that baby formula was much better than breast milk for children. Now the exact opposite is shown to be true.

Milk was recommended for coating the stomach and alleviating stomach ulcers. Now it is discouraged and has been found to aggravate ulcers.

Medical science stated that diet has absolutely no effect on disease or illness. Now we are told that diet has a huge effect on the prevention and cause of disease.

Medical science once had scientific evidence that the removing of tonsils and appendix improved health and should be done to virtually everyone. Now the medical community has reversed that theory.

Children with asthma were told to stay in enclosed pool areas because the humidity was good for their asthmatic condition. Now research suggests that the chlorine in the air from the pools actually aggravates and makes the asthma worse.

The most obvious example of all is the fact that there are thousands of drugs that have been approved by the FDA because they were scientifically proven to cure or prevent disease, in addition to having been touted as safe. Then, years later, they have been taken off the market because they had been newly proven to either not cure or prevent those diseases as originally thought, or those drugs were found to have such terribly adverse side effects that they are simply too dangerous for people to use."

Medical science has given us so much but we shouldn't presume that it's all facts. We should always keep an open mind and consider natural alternatives to find out what is better in reality, not in theory. Fanaticism is very dangerous as we need to know what is actually better for our health, so we don't live by discrepant theories.

American Dietetic Association views on veganism

Many doctors and health organizations have acknowledged that vegetarian diets can be a healthy way of life. In 2009 the **Academy of Nutrition and Dietetics** published the American Dietetic Association's (ADA) view that if a vegan diet was followed correctly it was very beneficial for us.[146] I have included a section of this article below:

"Appropriate Planned Vegetarian Diets Are Healthful, May Help in Disease Prevention and Treatment, Says American Dietetic Association

CHICAGO – The American Dietetic Association has released an updated position paper on vegetarian diets that concludes such diets, if well-planned, are healthful and nutritious for adults, infants, children and adolescents and can help prevent and treat chronic diseases including heart disease, cancer, obesity and diabetes.
ADA's position, published in the July issue of the Journal of the American Dietetic Association, represents the Association's official stance on vegetarian diets:
It is the position of the American Dietetic Association that appropriately planned vegetarian diets, including total vegetarian or vegan diets, are healthful, nutritionally adequate and may provide health benefits in the prevention and treatment of certain diseases. Well-planned vegetarian diets are appropriate for individuals during all stages of the life-cycle including pregnancy, lactation, infancy, childhood and adolescence and for athletes.
ADA's position and accompanying paper were written by Winston Craig, PhD, MPH, RD, professor and chair of the department of nutrition and wellness at Andrews University; and Reed Mangels, PhD, RD, nutrition advisor at the Vegetarian Resource Group, Baltimore, Md.

The revised position paper incorporates new topics and additional information on key nutrients for vegetarians, vegetarian diets in the life cycle and the use of vegetarian diets in prevention and treatment of chronic diseases. "Vegetarian diets are appropriate for all stages of the life cycle," according to ADA's position. "There are many reasons for the rising interest in vegetarian diets. The number of vegetarians in the United States is expected to increase over the next decade."

Vegetarian diets are often associated with health advantages including lower blood cholesterol levels, lower risk of heart disease, lower blood pressure levels and lower risk of hypertension and type 2 diabetes, according to ADA's position. "Vegetarians tend to have a lower body mass index and lower overall cancer rates. Vegetarian diets tend to be lower in saturated fat and cholesterol and have higher levels of dietary fiber, magnesium and potassium, vitamins C and E, folate, carotenoids, flavonoids and other phytochemicals. These nutritional differences may explain some of the health advantages of those following a varied, balanced vegetarian diet."

The position paper draws on results from ADA's evidence analysis process and information from the ADA Evidence Analysis Library to show vegetarian diets can be nutritionally adequate in pregnancy and result in positive maternal and infant health outcomes. Additionally, an evidence-based review showed a vegetarian diet is associated with a lower risk of death from ischemic heart disease.

A section in ADA's paper on vegetarian diets and cancer has been significantly expanded to provide details on cancer-protective factors in vegetarian diets.

An expanded section on osteoporosis includes roles of fruits, vegetables, soy products, protein, calcium, vitamins D and K and potassium in bone health. "Registered dietitians can provide information about key nutrients, modify vegetarian diets to meet the needs of those with dietary restrictions due to disease or allergies and supply guidelines to meet needs of clients in different areas of the life cycle," the authors said.

The American Dietetic Association is the world's largest organization of food and nutrition professionals. ADA is committed to improving the nation's health and advancing the profession of dietetics through research, education and advocacy."

Visit the American Dietetic Association at *www.eatright.org*.[147]"

An article published by the National Institutes of Health entitled *'Vegetarian Diets: What Are The Advantages?'*,[148] also supports adopting a vegetarian diet as a healthy way of life. The article explains that deficiencies in several nutrients like zinc, n-3 fatty acids and vitamin B12 can be found in a balanced vegetarian diet.

Future of Medical Sciences

There is no doubt as to the value of medical science both for the prevention and treatment of diseases. In our modern day society it is vital in accident and emergency cases. However, this does not mean that we should depend on this alone and solely look to doctors and drugs to guide the way. We should first ensure our body is strong enough to give us the best chance of fighting disease.

Medical science has a place in our society and we must continue to fund it so new cures can be found and our society continues to prosper in other areas.

The first step to strengthening our body's defenses is a healthy lifestyle, which is not possible without a healthy diet and good habits like regular exercise along with positive and happy thinking.

We cannot expect medical science to help us if we don't help ourselves first and break bad habits.

I do not agree with those that believe doctors would be without their job if we all became raw vegans. The most important purpose of funding medical science is to improve our health, so every open-minded doctor can feel assured that there are natural ways we can keep ourselves healthy without having to constantly visit them for every ailment or bad feeling we have.

The pressures of being a doctor are high due to the long hours worked and the responsibility. By keeping ourselves healthy through a natural diet, it lessens our chances of becoming sick thus alleviating some of the pressure on the medical profession. This enables doctors and scientists to have more time to research and provide better services for patients.

The continued research carried out by medical scientists to improve existing drugs and make them safe is vital. One example of this is anesthetic drugs, which previously had been very dangerous due to the many side effects. However, today they are much safer. Of course not using them at all would be ideal, for example, in some cases being hypnotized can be an alternative for anesthetic drugs[149].

Scientific tests based on raw vegans

Many health theories that are based on medical tests are often full of contradictions which do not provide any value for raw vegans, who have a completely different lifestyle in comparison with other patients.

A possible reason for this is that most medical experiences are done on sick people with unhealthy diets to enable certain tests to be carried out in order to prove certain theories. Medical science is supposed to help sick people while helping others to prevent diseases. If these experiments were based on completely healthy bodies and natural nutrition, the results would be very different.

Even with routine medical services, there are still many diagnostic errors, which pose significant problems in the medical world[150].

Humans have been consuming unhealthy and unnatural foods for centuries. This is bound to influence the conclusions reached by medical scientists.

Despite developments in medical science, we still do not have enough knowledge and there is too much conflicting information which cannot be useful for us, because we cannot accept any illusion as truth.

Most doctors expect all vegans to be deficient in iron and iodine but this is not so. Unfortunately despite the billions of dollars spent on advances in medical science we still cannot prevent certain deficiencies even in people who eat everything and have a common so-called "healthy diet". There are many meat-eaters who have an iron deficiency, so meat and animal products are not the answer.

But followers of a natural diet and especially those individuals, who have been raw vegans for several years, consume organic food as much as possible, exercise and have a balanced life, commonly do not have any deficiencies.

I believe it is necessary to repeat all medical tests and maybe redefine all standards using the example of raw veganism. We know that repeatable ability is one of the conditions for each credible experiment. By repeating all tests in a non-biased way, we will get clearer results.

I believe the true purpose of scientific experiments and research is not just to produce articles and papers, but to help the human race to achieve positive results in life by reaching perdurable health and merriment.

Brain food

Following a vegetarian diet can help to boost brain power. Many yoga masters and those that regularly perform mind exercises are vegetarian or vegan and recommend the diet to others as it helps boost the operation of the brain. In the science world, some great scientists are also vegetarian.

Since changing my diet and lifestyle I feel calmer and have a sense of peace as well as the noticeable improvement to my health. I can think clearer than ever before. Speaking to other raw vegans they have also expressed the same feelings since changing their diet.

A healthy diet, especially if it is based on natural foods, is very beneficial for your mental state mind. But, like other theories surrounding nutrition and health, there are some controversial ones surrounding the relationship between diet and the mind. Some scientists have claimed that cooking foods does increase the quality of that food for humans and helps the brain to develop as more energy is being extracted from the food which is then made available for the brain.

Some people profess that meat-eating improves the ability of our mind; while we know that the only energy source for the brain is glucose, which is found in most fruits.

Glucose is virtually the sole fuel for the human brain, except during prolonged starvation. The brain lacks fuel stores and hence requires a continuous supply of glucose. It consumes about 120g daily, which equals an energy input of about 420 kcal (1760 kJ), accounting for some 60% of the utilization of glucose by the whole body in the resting state.[151]

Frederic Patenaude, one of the most active raw food activists, talks about such theories in an article published on his blog entitled: '*Did We Adapt to Cooked Foods?*'[152] Patenaude agrees that extracting more energy from foods could help humans to increase the size of their brain but argues a fruit-based diet, which includes blended vegetables, can do just this as it eases the digestion process leaving more available calories to energize the body. A diet high in fat and protein with less fruit may make you feel less energized because fats and proteins are much harder to digest in comparison with natural simple sugars. Patenaude concludes that some incomplete theories on this subject can at least help us to become more curious about the truth and lead us to discover the mistakes in our diet.

A healthy and natural diet contains useful and necessary nutrients for the brain to function as well as reducing or even preventing the effects of age-related conditions, such as Alzheimer's or dementia. For this purpose, a healthy diet should contain enough amounts of antioxidants, which protect the body against free radicals. The useful nutrients for the brain are also useful for other organs of body as well, such as Omega 3 fatty acid, vitamin E and B vitamins.[153] Cooking destroys most of these nutrients so it may make it even harder to feed the brain, until the majority of the diet consists of fruit and vegetables.

We know that most of the vital energy of foods is destroyed by heating. Another problem is that cooked food is recognized by the body as a foreign invader, a threat to your health, so your body reacts to cooked food much the same way it does to bacteria, viruses and fungi in that it drastically increases its white blood cell count. White blood cells defend your body against toxins. Since the body recognizes cooked food as a toxin, it attacks it and tries to eliminate it. Eventually, sickness results because the body cannot eliminate the toxins fast enough. This process does not happen when you eat raw food because the body does not recognize raw food as a threat.[154]

It is logical to conclude that cooking at high temperatures is not compatible with the laws of nature which has evolved over millions of years. The human brain and its abilities have no such relation with food, because each great change in nature's evolution has taken thousands and even millions of years while cooking food before we consume it has only occurred for several thousand years.

Not only do raw vegan people feel a sense of well being, but also their mind powers have increased in most cases. This is provided they don't make any mistakes in their eating habits like eating too many grains or consuming the wrong food combinations, which can cause digestive difficulties and have negative effects on brain as well.

Raw foods can be beneficial not only in general, but also in emergency situations like accidents and other unwelcome events which may occur[155]. A good example of this is in the case of Tanya Alekseeva, who switched her diet to raw foods after surviving a near fatal car crash and numerous digestive problems. She healed and now she is a wellness coach[156].

Animals' natural food instincts and their intelligence

We should consider that intelligence exists in other animals and creatures, too. The intelligence of humans is just one form of intelligence and just because animals cannot invent computers doesn't mean they are not intelligent. Every creature has a different level of intelligence.

For example if a horse finds or is given a melon it will eat it in its entirety including the rind and seeds. The seeds of a melon contain some very useful minerals and anti-parasites, and its rind helps to improve digestion and prevent flatulence. This is completely compatible with the needs of the animal and the horse knows this instinctively. As humans we only know this on the basis of science and research.

Another example is when animals fast especially in winter during hibernation, which we know is very useful for body detoxification. Water fasting is recommended by many natural hygiene institutes as one of the best methods to heal certain illnesses. Animals benefit from the healing power of fasting while surviving when foods are not available to them.

Each creature wants to remain itself and reproduce another generation. Every plant or animal has some special instincts which help it during its life. This can also be counted as a kind of sagacity because every creature has its own role in nature which has to be completed. The intelligence of animals is far greater than humans used to think. For example, dolphins can communicate via echolation, while hyenas use smell-based networking sites. Even the marmoset monkeys have figured out how to have a polite conversation, something many humans still find hard to achieve[157]. So it's important to determine what we mean by the word intelligence.

Our brain and its potential

If we think of the special ingenuity of humans which helps him to invent new , then this is a positive and helpful intelligence. We know that each human uses only 6-7 % of his mind, we don't know much about the rest of it. There are different theories about the rest of our mind power. Some theories relate to the so-called Golden Age in human history which suggests that there were developed civilizations in ancient times which were completely destroyed and our civilization is possibly based on what remained from the sciences of this age.

In Greek and Roman mythology, the Golden Age was the first Age of the world, where humans lived in a Utopia of ideal happiness. It then degenerates i.e. Silver, Bronze, Heroic and Iron[158].

Some religions believe that humans "fell down" from their original position through ignorance and unconsciousness, which they describe as a so-called sin. Taking these beliefs into consideration is acceptable but it seems obvious that humans could have had a much better life than what we experience today. Greed, bad thoughts and wrong deeds are making us humans miserable. One could argue that consuming cooked foods lowered our intelligence levels as we know it is not very beneficial for our body and thus, it is not so strange to conclude that eating cooked food may not be beneficial for the mind also.

Here the question is: Is it really worth destroying our health with harmful meats and cooked food for the sake of a theory that meat is supposed to be useful for the human brain?

A balanced life is very important, and fortunately, with a healthy body we can use our brain much better. We do not need to destroy our body with saturated fats and carcinogenic chemical materials found in meat, while we are not even certain that meat is really useful for the brain. This seems more likely to be a myth than a fact.

The mutual relationship between body and mind is really very obvious, while we don't know everything about it yet. What we eat can affect our mind and what we think can also affect our physical health. Therefore, we are responsible for what we eat and what we think. This matters more than unproven and incomplete theories.

Organic agriculture

Our agricultural system up until now has not shown itself as the perfect system in terms of providing sufficient and healthy food to feed the world; it needs to change. We simply cannot sustain the quality in our food supply if we don't change our agricultural system. Soil weakness is caused by different pollutants, excessive deforestation, acidic rain and too much cattle grazing. This can cause a shortage of plant food and can also cause different deficiencies in our body. When quality is sacrificed only for quantity, we can't expect the results to be good.

Chemical fertilizers harm the soil, water, plants and the human body.[159] Fruits and vegetables grown with the aid of chemical fertilizers decay sooner than organic fruits and vegetables. They are also usually less effective in helping to alkalize the body in comparison with natural and organic plant foods. Most pesticide residue on fruits and vegetables are also acidic, so given that the human body should have an alkaline PH of about 7.3 to 7.6 to remain healthy, the chemical acidic compounds which we eat every day can damage our health over time.[160]

Natural fertilizers such as animal dung or plant compost are much better than chemical fertilizers, because not only are they better for the environment, but they contain useful bacteria and other live micro-organisms, which have a very important role in strengthening soil and help to increase the quality of the crop, while chemical fertilizers kill many useful micro-organisms when they are used regularly and in large amounts.[161]

Natural fertilizers such as animal dung contain a much better balance of minerals than chemical fertilizers. Food grown using artificial fertilizers are not as tasty as natural organic foods and also have fewer nutrients in comparison to organic foods. Natural animal dung is one of the benefits of animals so we shouldn't just assume that God has created them only to be eaten by other animals.

Many people think that organic agriculture cannot produce enough food to feed the world alone as the world's population continues to increase. While some studies do not support the idea of a completely organic agricultural system because of the increasing demand for food, it still supports the idea of a hybrid approach[162]. While research, such as that from the Soil Association, says there is now evidence to suggest that a switch to organic farming in the Global South could even increase production[163].

The Food and Agriculture Organization of the United Nations explains the importance of food security:

"Food security is not only a question of the ability to produce food, but also of the ability to access food. Global food production is more than enough to feed the global population; the problem is getting it to the people who need it. In market-marginalized areas, organic farmers can increase food production by managing local resources without having to rely on external inputs or food distribution systems over which they have little control and/or access."[164]

A healthy diet even with non-organic foods

Unfortunately the majority of our food is poisoned with different chemicals, but as a raw vegan this does not mean that because I cannot always access organic foods my diet isn't beneficial. Almost all raw vegans (including me) have benefitted from this diet even if it includes non-organic fruits. When I started following my diet in Iran, organic fruit was not available to me yet still my severe headaches and other health problems went after I switched to a raw vegan diet.

If we want to eat only organic foods our diet could become very limited and this could cause other problems so we shouldn't be fanatical about the issue. However, we should be aware of what we consume and support organic food producers as much as possible to help change ourselves and the world. This is a long-term aim that we have to be aware of and responsible for.

If more people changed their eating habits there would be more food available, so by choosing a wise and balanced lifestyle we can hope that our food supply problems could be solved sooner.

But for now, there are some tips to improve our diet such as eating fruit that is in season as they have fewer pesticides on them and eating fruit that is ripe and ready to eat. Sometimes conventionally grown fruits can be better than the organic ones, for example, a ripe conventionally grown mango is better to eat than an organic unripe mango and actually tastes better. Also sweet mango flesh is protected by its thick skin from pesticides. Still, you'll want to rinse under water before cutting open.

Other examples of fruits and vegetables which are safe to buy non organic include[165]:

Avocados which have thick skins that protect the fruit from any pesticide build-up. Look for avocados that are unripe and firm to the squeeze; they'll ripen nicely on your kitchen counter in a couple of days. Always store at room temperature. Although you'll be using only the flesh of the avocado, it's always a good idea to rinse them before you slice them open.

Pineapple also has a tough skin which protects the fruit from pesticide residue. As with all your produce, you should rinse the pineapple before cutting.

Sweet corn may take a lot of fertilizer to grow, but you're unlikely to end up with any pesticides on the kernels. Make sure you select those that are not genetically modified organisms (GMO).

Cabbage doesn't require a lot of chemical fertilizers to grow. Look for cabbage heads with tight leaves and make sure the outer leaves are shiny and crisp. Savoy is the exception to this rule, as it forms a looser head and the leaves grow crinkly naturally. You'll want to avoid any with leaves that show signs of yellowing. Bok Choy should have deep green leaves with their stems being a crisp-looking white. Discard the outer leaves of a cabbage before using. You can wash and spin most cabbage leaves just like you do salad greens.

The enjoyment of following a healthy diet

Some meat eaters think that only fleshy, cooked foods are tasty and all raw plant foods are unsavory. Some believe that raw food eaters torture themselves to remain healthy. But in fact all the views we have are just personal views based on our experiences so are not necessarily the absolute perfect truth.

Meat eaters have fallen into the habit of eating meat after being force fed it over and over again, until they become accustomed to such food; while raw foods, especially fruits, we immediately find delicious. If a raw plant or vegetable isn't savory for us but we still want to eat it anyhow, we can mix it with some compatible vegetables to make it more flavorsome. This is much healthier than cooking food in the hope of making it taste better.

There are so many vegan and raw food recipes which are often more diverse than many meat recipes. It just takes a little time and effort for us to get used to a raw vegan diet while we can enjoy its health benefits immediately.

When you switch to a vegan diet the feeling of wellbeing is another reason why this way of eating is enjoyable. You are eating an eco-friendly diet and doing so much more than just trying to fill your belly.

Animal flesh is not human food

A little after starting my veganism journey, I saw a report on a television health news show called What's Good For You[166] which showed researchers in Australia who were trying to find a way of improving the taste of meat to make it appealing for older people who no longer found it appetizing. They did this by adding spices and other chemical materials. There are many useless experiments carried out in the name of "science" and a lot of money spent in vain on such actions every year. Such so-called "research" has no benefit for humans, except to make money for junk food markets in the worst possible way.

When we get older and no longer enjoy the taste of meat it just shows us that eating animal corpses isn't natural for humans. Yet all people, young or old, will enjoy the taste of fresh fruits and vegetables because these are natural foods for humans. You don't see experiments to improve the taste of dates or bananas to make them appealing for older people.

New recipes are constantly being introduced to improve the taste of meat because animal carcasses are not tasty and are not our natural foods, so we have to use spices, herbs and other foods to make it more palatable.

Start changing your lifestyle

As you come to the end of the first part of my book I hope you have learnt the most important principles of a healthy lifestyle, backed by scientific and experimental details. If you are not a vegan/raw vegan, your diet is not very healthy and you want to change, I want to congratulate you for wanting to make the change.

In the first part of my book, which focused on nutrition, I have endeavored to provide enough information to stop people from making any mistakes when changing their diet.

How you change your diet is up to you but by making some changes to improve your diet, based on what you have read so far, will be of great benefit.

If others can do it, so can you.

In the next part of my book, you will learn why it is important to change your diet on a global scale.

So, good luck with your life journey.

Chapter 2: Healthy Lifestyle and the Economy

Economic problems are undoubtedly one of the biggest issues facing our world today and no country is immune. Whether a country's financial hardship is due to natural disasters, over consumption or corrupt governments, they all have negative repercussions on society.

The economy is an important part of every society. Each economic crisis will have a negative effect on the society surrounding it. A person's financial hardship will have repercussions on many aspects on that person's life including their nutrition and health.

Economic difficulties often force people to resort to buying cheap unhealthy food which makes them even more vulnerable to disease. People spend money on useless cheap food, get sick and then have to spend more money on treatment, whilst their sickness reduces their working efficiency impacting on the economy further. The irony being that person has to work more to cover their medical and insurance costs despite being sick.

Producing animal products is much more expensive than producing plant foods because more natural resources are required. This is explained in more detail in the John Vidal's article '*10 ways vegetarianism can help save the planet*[167]'. In it he writes:

"Nearly 30% of the available ice-free surface area of the planet is now used by livestock, or for growing food for those animals.

One billion people go hungry every day, but livestock now consumes the majority of the world's crops. A Cornell University study in 1997 found that around 13m hectares of land in the US were used to grow vegetables, rice, fruit, potatoes and beans, but 302m were used for livestock. The problem is that farm animals are inefficient converters of food to flesh. Broiler chickens are the best, needing around 3.4kg to produce 1kg of flesh, but pigs need 8.4kg for that kilo. Other academics have calculated that if the grain fed to animals in western countries were consumed directly by people instead of animals, we could feed at least twice as many people – and possibly far more – as we do now."

A diet of meat, milk and dairy is not cheap while a raw vegan diet is not only cheaper but better for our health.

It is true that some meat can be cheap but I would like to include a quote from the article by Abigail Geer entitled '*The True Cost of Meat: Demystifying Agricultural Subsidies*[168]', which explains why buying some meat cuts can sometimes be cheaper than buying fruit.

"One of the most important factors affecting national and global food supplies is the amount of money which governments pay out in subsidies to farmers. Currently this is heavily weighted towards animal agriculture, making the cost of meat artificially low. Your tax money is paying for farmers to use and abuse these animals, and it's making it an affordable business model when in fact the real cost of producing meat would leave the livestock industry making a net loss. Something has to be awry when a chicken's life is reduced to a price tag, and when that price tag is less than what it costs to buy a pack of strawberries, you have to start asking how and why. If the government were to stop paying out huge sums of money to animal farmers and redistribute these funds to those wishing to grow fruits, vegetables and crops for human consumption, many of the world's food issues would disappear (along with the environmental and animal rights issues too)."

A major part of our taxes is spent on producing meat, which not only is unnecessary for us but also causes many health issues and is detrimental to our economy and environment. This is a true waste of money.

In *MEATONOMIC$'* author David Robinson Simon's article '*10 Things I Wish All Americans Knew About The Meat and Dairy Industries*', he explains the true cost of eating meat[169]:

"In a creepy, Big-Brotherish tactic straight out of a sci-fi movie, the federal government uses catchy slogans to get people to buy more meat and dairy.

Each year, USDA-managed programs spend $550 million to bombard Americans with slogans like these urging us to buy more animal foods. Although people in every age group already eat more animal protein than recommended, and far more than our forebears did, these promotional programs are shockingly effective at making us buy even more. Each marketing buck spent boosts sales by an average of $8, for an annual total of an extra $4.6 billion in government-backed sales of meat, dairy, and eggs.

Americans eat more meat per person than any other people on earth and we're paying the price in doctor bills.

At 200 pounds of meat per person per year, our high meat consumption is hurting our national health. Hundreds of clinical studies in the past several decades show that consumption of meat and dairy, especially at the high levels seen in this country, can cause cancer, diabetes, heart disease, and a host of other diseases. Thus, Americans have twice the obesity rate, twice the diabetes rate, and nearly three times the cancer rate as the rest of the world. Eating loads of meat isn't the only reason people develop these diseases, but it's a major factor.

There's no sustainable way to raise animal foods to meet the world's growing demand.

Two acres of rain forest are cleared each minute to raise cattle or crops to feed them. 35,000 miles of American rivers are polluted with animal waste. We're watching a real-time, head-on collision between the world's huge demand for animal foods and the reality of scarce resources. It takes dozens of times more water and five times more land to produce animal protein than equal amounts of plant protein. Unfortunately, even "green" alternatives like raising animals locally, organically, or on pastures can't overcome the basic math: the resources just don't exist to keep feeding the world animal foods at the level it wants.

American governments spend $38 billion each year to subsidize meat and dairy, but only 0.04% of that ($17 million) to subsidize fruits and vegetables.

The federal government's Dietary Guidelines urge us to eat more fruits and vegetables and less cholesterol-rich food (that is, meat and dairy). Yet like a misguided parent giving a kid cotton candy for dinner, state and federal governments get it backwards by giving buckets of cash to animal agriculture while providing almost no help to those raising fruits and vegetables."

An article published on the Physicians Committee for Responsible Medicine's (PCRM) website explains the cost of feeding animals and the effect on food prices overall[170]:

"Although the "Dietary Guidelines for Americans" call for reducing the intake of saturated fat and cholesterol, federal subsidies favor the production of meat and dairy products that are the principal sources of these hazardous components.

Much of the corn and soybeans grown in the United States, which together received more than $96 billion in subsidies over the last 15 years, is used for animal feed.

Changes in the cost of feed grains are reflected in changes in food prices at the retail level, although the precise impact depends on the proportion of grain input in the final product. The Center for Agricultural and Rural Development of Iowa State University estimated that a 30 percent change in the price of feed grain would change "egg prices by 8.1 percent, poultry prices by 5.1 percent, pork prices by 4.5 percent, beef prices by 4.1 percent, and milk prices by 2.7 percent."

For most livestock production operations, feed represents a significant portion of input costs. Between 1997 and 2005, large livestock producers saved an estimated $3.9 billion annually—nearly $35 billion in total—due to the reduced cost of feed containing subsidy-supported corn and soybeans.

According to an economic analysis by Elanor Starmer and Timothy Wise of Tufts University, "U.S. policies have made industrial livestock operations appear more cost-efficient than they would if feed were properly valued in the marketplace. They also suggest that taxpayers and farm families have, in effect, been subsidizing factory farms' feed purchases.""

The importance of our health during economic hardship

If we are faced with economic issues, the healthier we are the more able we are to cope with such pressures. Unfortunately for many people facing such stresses, the opposite is more common. It is often the case that a person's perturbation of their economic situation has a negative effect on their diet.

Health; the first step to peace

Trillions of dollars are spent every year fighting heart disease and cancer, which can be prevented with a healthy diet and lifestyle. Imagine what we could do with this huge amount of money which is spent on treating diseases, not even trying to tackle the root cause, just providing treatments. It is estimated that almost one trillion (1,000 billion) US dollars is spent annually just on treating heart disease around the world. This is almost equal to the total value of the three big technology companies: Apple, Google and Microsoft. So imagine if we can reduce disease and spend this money on industry or agriculture instead of wasting it on maladies.

To be a healthy person means the following;

Healthy body = Healthy mind

Healthy mind = Healthy person

Healthy Person = More efficient

More efficient = Better economic development

Better economic development = More opportunities for industrial development

More opportunities for industry development = More advanced world

More advanced world = Discovering better ways to sustain our environment

Healthier environment = More welfare in society

More welfare in society = More chance for peace

More peace = More happiness

More happiness = The real life

How veganism can help the economy and society

Meat is expensive and wastes valuable resources to produce. As explained in Section 1 (Veganism and Health), meat is very harmful for the human body and can make us sick pushing up the cost of healthcare.

With raw veganism there is no need to worry about a lack of food as there will always be more food available than people need. Vegetative foods are more economically sound than animal products as their price, on average, is about one third of animal products. In comparison animal foods, especially organic, are more expensive. This is because a farm is needed to grow an animal to use its meat or milk, while the food resulting from that animal is less than one tenth of the amount of plant foods which could be gained from that farm. We also need to factor in the price of collecting and storing foods for cattle in winter, the cost of preventing and treating diseases and finally, the cost of running fridges to keep meat[171]. Saving and storing meat is usually more difficult than plant foods and needs advanced technology.

Cattle are not immune to disease so when this occurs the affected animals have to be destroyed forfeiting all the money spent on keeping and raising it. Premature cattle deaths have declined over the years due to advances in science. This has led to an enormous amount of money being spent on the maintenance and vaccination of animals which grow in an unnatural environment. Diseases such as foot and mouth and mad cow disease are occurring because of unnatural genetic changes, hormone injections, chemical drugs and artificial insemination to force animals to give birth several times in one year.

Perhaps it seems hard to believe, but eating meat wastes our natural resources while millions of people suffer from malnutrition and millions of them perish every year.

If all people on earth were vegan, it would be possible to feed three to five times more than the current number of inhabitants. Herbal foods are not only good for our health but also very advantageous from an economic perspective.

Raw Veganism is the best diet economically

Veganism helps our economy and environment, but raw veganism can be even more effective.

 As Arshavir Ter-Hovanessian's wrote in his book '*Raw-Eating: The philosophy of nutrition and health*' back in 1976 we can never run out of natural foods. He said:

"If so-called "civilized" people don't destroy natural foods with fire thoughtlessly, it's possible to nourish five times more than the current population of the world with these available foods.

The "civilized" people annihilate eighty percent of foods (which they get from the soil) by fire, and after, they talk about a "lack of food".

If people stop using dead foods they don't diminish anything and they get rid of unnatural and poisonous materials which cause many diseases. These statements seem unbelievable for dead food eaters, but it's the truth. If a dead food eater eats one bunch of grapes per week, this amount of grapes and a small amount of other foods cells which remain alive after eating dead foods feeds him and keeps him alive. This shows us just how much value natural foods have. Some scientists try to produce artificial and compressed foods to save people from cooking, they don't observe that nature did this already with foods like almonds, wheat and walnuts. If everyone kept a handful of these foods in their pocket they could happily work all day requiring no other food.

An Iranian worker spends half of his income buying bread every day, but his wife and children are still hungry, always sick and weak, while if this worker buys only half a kilo of wheat (every day) for his family, he can give them enough to eat and keep them healthy. This food is the work of our great creator (God) which most people haven't yet discovered.

Now there are some nations which suffer from a lack of food and are near starvation but with just one announcement from that nation's Ministry of Health stating that cooking is wrong and dangerous, would be enough for those nations to remain secure from every misfortune.

If in ancient times, soldiers surrounding cities and forts had rationed raw wheat instead of bread, their resistance time could have been longer and as a result, the map of the world would look a lot different today.

Some people ask me if we don't eat "baked" foods what should we eat. In their view, food means something that has been completely killed in the kitchen. But those who want to live a healthy and long life should firstly forget that there is any cooked food in this world, secondly they should see what all animals eat, from an ant to an elephant so they can understand the real value of all vegetables and fruits which they have access to. "Nutrition experts" leave people confused about food as they give them contradictory information."

So changing our diet to vegan or raw vegan has an undeniable effect on the economy because if an individual gets his or her food needs from worthwhile herbal resources instead of wasting money on meat, costs will decrease, our health will improve and we will have more money to help change our life for the better.

Eating meat is harmful for our body and the cost of producing it is very expensive made more so by government subsides[172] which take away vital funds from other areas such as developing agriculture and building more schools.

Our diet and its effects on global warming costs

Research done by the Netherlands Environmental Assessment discovered that changing the diet of the world's population would decrease the cost of fighting global warming. The findings were as follows:

Cost of decreasing greenhouse gases in the atmosphere until the year 2050, is 40 trillion dollars.

Decreasing meat consumption at a global level will decrease 50% of the total cost of solving global warming.

Stopping using meats at a global level can decrease 70% of total costs.[173]

The vegan industry

I often get asked what would become of certain industries if everyone became vegan, such as farmers, fishermen and non vegetarian restaurant owners.

Firstly, everybody can change their job and choose an occupation which is profitable whilst moral and enjoyable for that person, too.

With an increasing number of people becoming vegan, it is necessary to develop agriculture further, especially organic agriculture. Requests for natural and organic food increases every day, thereupon, a producer of processed foods (like cold cuts and sausage) can be changed to a producer of organic foods to fulfill this demand.

One man who changed his job after becoming vegan was Howard F. Lyman who was a great cowman. He was diagnosed with spine cancer and after he successfully underwent surgery which had a success rate of one in a million, he became vegan and changed his job. He wrote and published the book 'Mad Cowboy' about this subject. He endeavored to invite people to veganism and exposed certain acts taking place in animal husbandry, like making powder from the carcasses of animals and mixing it with cattle feed.

In veganism there is no spite against certain workers; the point is to create an ideal world where all people are happy and healthy.

Making veganism more popular can end starvation so there will be no hungry children and we can all enjoy the worthy gift of health.

Chapter 3: Healthy Lifestyle and the Environment

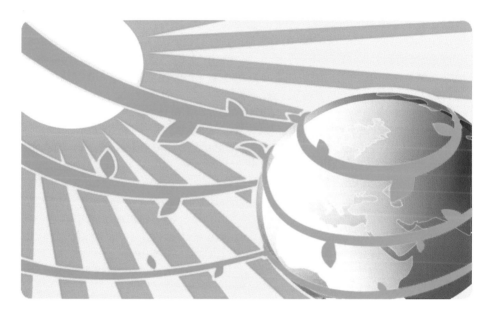

In today's world we face many serious environmental issues that have direct and indirect effects on human health. Unfortunately serious actions to rectify the situation haven't been taken because more attention has been paid to the financial implications of dealing with these issues, instead of looking after the environment in which we all live.

Our damaged and polluted environment is the cause of most diseases and famines.

Industrial activities and animal husbandries produce huge amounts of trash and paying little attention to recycling and cultural poverty in many parts of the world make it more complex to revive the environment. But this is a matter which we cannot ignore because if the environment is destroyed, we will be destroyed too.

PROTECTING THE EARTH

The US-based group Vegan Outreach explains on its website[174] why raising cattle for food is detrimental to the environment.

"When carbon dioxide, methane and nitrous oxide are released into the air they blanket the earth, trapping heat inside the atmosphere. This is known as the greenhouse effect, and it keeps our planet at a temperature at which life can thrive. The problem is the massive increase in the output of these and other greenhouse gases since industrialization has caused the effect to intensify.

"The livestock sector is a major player, responsible for 18 percent of greenhouse gas emissions measured in CO_2 equivalent. This is a higher share than transport." (Transport causes 13.5%) - The United Nations FAO

A University of Chicago study comparing a typical US meat-based diet with a vegan diet found that the 'typical' US diet generates the equivalent of nearly 1.5 tons more carbon dioxide per person per year than a vegan diet. The authors of the study concluded that it would be more environmentally effective to go vegan than to switch to a petrol electric hybrid car.

The felling of forests to grow food for the exploding population of cattle, pigs and chickens, results in fewer trees to absorb carbon dioxide and is a major contributor to global warming.

The following findings were compiled from the executive summary of Livestock's Long Shadow[175]: Environmental Issues and Options, a 2006 report published by the United Nations Food and Agriculture Organization:

Climate change: With rising temperatures, rising sea levels, melting icecaps and glaciers, shifting ocean currents and weather patterns, climate change is the most serious challenge facing the human race. The livestock sector is a major player, responsible for 18 percent of greenhouse gas emissions measured in CO_2 equivalent.... Livestock are also responsible for almost two-thirds (64 percent) of anthropogenic ammonia emissions, which contribute significantly to acid rain and acidification of ecosystems.

Water: The livestock sector is a key player in increasing water use, accounting for over 8 percent of global human water use, mostly for the irrigation of feed crops. It is probably the largest sectoral source of water pollution, contributing to eutrophication, "dead" zones in coastal areas, degradation of coral reefs, human health problems, emergence of antibiotic resistance and many others. The major sources of pollution are from animal waste, antibiotics and hormones, chemicals from tanneries, fertilizers and pesticides used for feed crops, and sediments from eroded pastures.

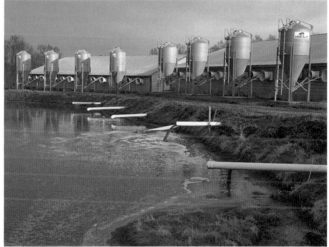

Hog farm waste lagoons in Georgia

Photo credit: courtesy of USDA

Land degradation: Expansion of livestock production is a key factor in deforestation, especially in Latin America where the greatest amount of deforestation is occurring – 70 percent of previous forested land in the Amazon is occupied by pastures, and feed crops cover a large part of the remainder.

Biodiversity: Indeed, the livestock sector may well be the leading player in the reduction of biodiversity, since it is the major driver of deforestation, as well as one of the leading drivers of land degradation, pollution, climate change, overfishing, sedimentation of coastal areas and facilitation of invasions by alien species."

For more information, see the Media Release and Full Report of FAO.[176]

According to the EPA's article *'Animal Waste: What's the Problem?'*177:

"The growing scale and concentration of animal feeding operations (AFOs) has contributed to negative environmental and human health impacts. Pollution associated with AFOs degrades the quality of waters, threatens drinking water sources, and may harm air quality.

By definition, AFOs produce large amounts of waste in small areas. For example, a single dairy cow produces approximately 120 pounds of wet manure per day. Estimates equate the waste produced per day by one dairy cow to that of 20–40 humans per day.

Manure, and wastewater containing manure, can severely harm river and stream ecosystems. Manure contains ammonia which is highly toxic to fish at low levels. Increased amounts of nutrients, such as nitrogen and phosphorus, from AFOs can cause algal blooms which block waterways and deplete oxygen as they decompose. This can kill fish and other aquatic organisms, devastating the entire aquatic food chain.

Millions of gallons of liquefied feces and urine seeped into the environment from collapsed, leaking or overflowing storage lagoons, and flowed into rivers, streams, lakes, wetlands and groundwater. Hundreds of manure spills have killed millions of fish.

Intensive pig farms have made the air so unbearable in some rural communities that some residents must wear masks while outdoors[178] and made some people sick. Poultry and pig waste has contributed to the growth of pathogenic organisms in waterways, which have poisoned humans and killed millions of fish. From 1995 to 1997, more than forty animal waste spills killed 10.6 million fish."

It's clear that we need to act now if we are to save our environment from further damage, damage that cannot be rectified at a later date. We all have our part to play, it surrounds us all and we are all responsible[179].

Meat eating and global warming

The industrial activities of man produce 49% of greenhouse gases, the most important gases in relation to the greenhouse effect. However, animal husbandry on its own is responsible for producing 51% of greenhouse gases.

An article which featured in the British newspaper the Independent stated that according to an article published by a respected US think-tank the Worldwatch Institute, two World Bank environmental advisers claim that instead of 18 per cent of global emissions being caused by meat, the true figure is 51 per cent.

The article goes on to say:

"They claim that United Nation's figures have severely underestimated the greenhouse gases caused by tens of billions of cattle, sheep, pigs, poultry and other animals in three main areas: methane, land use and respiration.

Their findings – which are likely to prompt fierce debate among academics – come amid increasing calls from climate change experts for people to eat less meat. In the 19-page report, Robert Goodland, a former lead environmental adviser to the World Bank, and Jeff Anhang, a current adviser, suggest that domesticated animals cause 32 billion tons of carbon dioxide equivalent (CO2e), more than the combined impact of industry and energy. The accepted figure is 18 per cent, taken from a landmark UN report in 2006, Livestock's Long Shadow.[180]

Scientists are concerned about livestock's exhalation of methane, a potent greenhouse gas. Cows and other ruminants emit 37 per cent of the world's methane."[181]

A cow, on average, releases between 70 and 120 kg of methane per year. Methane is a greenhouse gas like carbon dioxide (CO2) but the negative effect on the climate is 23 times higher than the effect of CO2. Therefore the release of about 100 kg of methane per year for each cow is equivalent to about 2,300 kg of CO2 per year.

To compare the value of 2,300 kg of CO2, the same amount of CO2 is generated by burning 1,000 liters of petrol. With a car using eight liters of petrol per 100 km, you could drive 12,500 km per year (7,800 miles per year). Worldwide, there are about 1.5 billion cows and bulls. All ruminants (animals which regurgitate food and re-chew it) worldwide emit about two billion metric tons of CO2-equivalents per year. In addition, the clearing of tropical forests and rainforests to get more grazing land and farm land is responsible for an extra 2.8 billion metric tons of CO2 emissions per year.

A Japanese study showed that producing a kilogram of beef leads to the emission of greenhouse gases with a global warming potential equivalent to 36.4 kilograms of CO2. It also releases fertilizing compounds equivalent to 340 grams of sulfur dioxide and 59 grams of phosphate, and consumes 169 mega joules of energy. In other words, a kilogram of beef is responsible for the equivalent of the amount of CO2 emitted by the average European car every 250 kilometers, and burns enough energy to light a 100-watt bulb for nearly 20 days.[182]

As methane has 23-25 times more potential than carbon dioxide for contributing to global warming, reducing our meat consumption is the first and most important step to stop global warming. However a study in 2009 by the NASA Goddard Institute for Space Studies, has found methane is 33 times more damaging if the effects of interaction with other airborne pollutants is included.[183]

This is just one of the harms of fostering billions of animals for our consumption but if we add fire and deforestation to create cattle runs, then we will understand the depth of tragedy. Forests are the lungs of the earth so by destroying them it becomes harder to solve our environmental issues.[184]

According to PBL Netherlands Environmental Assessment Agency:
"Reducing global meat consumption would reduce greenhouse gas emissions and cut the costs of climate policy substantially. This is the result of a PBL study published in Climatic Change. Apart from a reduction in methane and N2O emissions, vast agricultural areas would become unused, mostly as a result of reduced cattle grazing, and could take up large amounts of carbon. Shifting worldwide to a healthy low-meat diet would reduce the costs of stabilizing greenhouse gases at 450 ppm CO2 eq. by more than 50%."[185]

Other harms of animal factory farming for the environment

The following explains further why animal factory farming is not good for our environment[186]:

Drinking too much water

Eat a steak or a chicken and you are effectively consuming the water that the animal has needed to live and grow. Vegetarian author John Robbins calculates it takes 60, 108, 168, and 229 pounds of water to produce one pound of potatoes, wheat, maize and rice respectively. But a pound of beef needs around 9,000 liters – or more than 20,000 lbs of water. Equally, it takes nearly 1,000 liters of water to produce one liter of milk. A broiler chicken, by contrast, is far more efficient, producing the same amount of meat as a cow on just 1,500 liters. Pigs are some of the thirstiest animals. An average-sized North American pig farm with 80,000 pigs needs nearly 75 million gallons of fresh water a year. A large one, which might have one million or more pigs, may need as much as a city. Farming, which uses 70% of water available to humans, is already in direct competition for water with cities. But as demand for meat increases, so there will be less available for both crops and drinking. Rich but water-stressed countries such as Saudi Arabia, Libya, the Gulf States and South Africa believe it makes sense to grow food in poorer countries to conserve their water resources, and are now buying or leasing millions of hectares of Ethiopia and elsewhere to provide their food. Every cow fattened in the Gambella state in southern Ethiopia and exported to Abu Dhabi or Britain is taking the pressure off water supplies back home but increasing it elsewhere.

Spoiling the oceans

Most summers between 13,000-20,000 sq km of sea at the mouth of the Mississippi becomes a dead zone, caused when vast quantities of excess nutrients from animal waste, factory farms, sewage, nitrogen compounds and fertilizer are swept down the mighty river. This causes algal blooms which take up all the oxygen in the water to the point where little can live. Nearly 400 dead zones ranging in size from one to over 70,000sq km have now been identified, from the Scandinavian fjords to the South China Sea. Animal farming is not the only culprit, but it is one of the worst.

Air quality

Anyone who has lived close to a large factory farm knows the smells can be extreme. Aside from greenhouse gases such as methane and carbon dioxide, cows and pigs produce many other polluting gases. Global figures are unavailable but in the US, livestock and animal feed crops are responsible for 37% of pesticide use, more than half of all the antibiotics manufactured and a third of the nitrogen and phosphorous in fresh water. Nearly two thirds of the manmade ammonia – a major contributor to acid rain – is also generated by livestock. In addition, the concentrated factory farming of animals contributes to ozone pollution.

A plant-based and environmentally friendly diet

A plant-based diet and healthy lifestyle is very effective in reviving the environment.

In 2009 researchers from the Netherlands Environmental Assessment Agency published their projections of the greenhouse gas consequences if we were to eat less meat, no meat, or no animal products at all. Researchers predicted that universal veganism would reduce agriculture-related carbon emissions by 17 percent, methane emissions by 24 percent, and nitrous oxide emissions by 21 percent by 2050. Universal vegetarianism would result in similarly impressive reductions in greenhouse gas emissions. What's more researchers found that worldwide vegetarianism or veganism would achieve these gains at a much lower cost than a purely energy-focused intervention involving carbon taxes and renewable energy technology.[187]

Veganism is the best and simplest way to protect the earth as well as being better for our health and the economy.

We should not forget that it's not only humans who have a right to live in a healthy environment, but animals also. All animals live their lives on earth and then die without damaging their surroundings while humans cause the extinction of certain types of animals and other critters through their actions. Man breeds animals for food using artificial insemination and hormone injections while the whole process pollutes our environment. It wastes an enormous amount of money and energy to create harmful food not to mention the torture which the animals suffer through the process.

Nature's delicate balance

Bounteous forests are destroyed so soy and corn farms can be established to nourish cattle while rivers and seas are overfished. Yet millions of people are still hungry and sick. But if plant-based diets became more popular there is no need for fishing or ruthless animal husbandry and nature will have a chance to recover. A plant-based diet will nourish more people as there won't be a need to use most of the crops grown for animal feed. In the US 80% of corn and at least 50% of soy grown goes directly to animal feed[188].

It's clear that a plant-based diet is the best solution for the environment. For me, it's very hard to imagine that a person wants to eat meat with avidity and voracity after researching its effects on our health, economy and environment.

Chapter 4: Natural Lifestyle, Society and Humanity

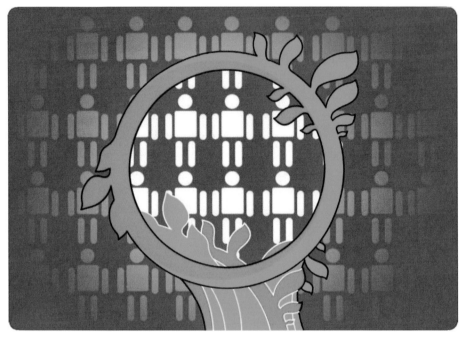

The benefits of a natural diet in terms of health, the economy, and our environment have already been explained so in this section I will be taking a closer look at the effects of a natural diet on the way humans behave in society.

If we all adopted a healthier diet, it would lead to a healthier environment and improve our economic situation. This would undoubtedly have a beneficial effect on our mental health; we'd be happier and behave better towards each other. The need to fight and start wars would be reduced because when we all have what we need there is no need to fight. It would no longer be necessary to forget our lives for the sake of one more dollar.

If man can invent and achieve what they have done so far despite the state of our world, imagine what can be accomplished if basic issues, such as supplying all that we need with the resources we have, was resolved.

Our modern world

Developments in technology have provided many benefits in terms of making people's daily lives a lot simpler. It has also made huge amounts of money for a small number of people, while polluting the environment.

Most scientists and inventors, who rely on and help to move technology forward, are humanitarian and kind-hearted people who just want to help others. But unfortunately our governing systems have ensured that technology has resulted in the oppression of people while making money for a small minority.

Money is not bad in itself, but it depends on our intention. It's a system which was invented to make trading easier. Now in this world, almost no one can live without money. It's necessary to have enough money and even have more than enough, but we must ensure that our income doesn't damage others.

How bad habits and sickness affect our fate

Bad habits such as drinking expensive alcoholic drinks instead of water or smoking cigars, marijuana, and cocaine instead of breathing fresh air all has a detrimental effect on society. Large amounts of money have to be spent to treat us when we get sick as a result of these bad habits.

We should also be aware that a sick person doesn't only hurt himself, but also hurts the family and friends around him or her. So everyone has to be responsible for their own health as much as possible. Of course there are special circumstances such as an accident or sudden event which can damage our health and are out of our control, but what we eat and our lifestyle is completely within our control.

Natural lifestyle, justice and humanity

Following a natural lifestyle provides a good opportunity for the mental and moral growth of society which can solve basic problems forever. Nature has ensured that we have access to the healthiest and most delicious foods. A wise person uses these blessings of nature and endeavors to achieve his/her wishes and well-being without damaging anything else.

There are a great many lucky people in this world that have had successful lives and have enjoyed their time as much as possible, but unfortunately, the number of successful people is very few in comparison with unsuccessful and unlucky people.

The cause of why only a few people were/are successful is the injustice in the world which was always an obstacle for clever people. Unfortunately, many talented people who had great potential to be successful but have remained disappointed and perished futilely.

Now imagine if suitable facilities were available for every person on earth to realize their talents and reach their potential, and imagine how many elite and capable people there would be in society. This is the true meaning of humanity. We should not forget others, because we are all the same in origin, and we all have the right to have a good life.

Making life easier

Adopting a natural diet means little time is spent on preparing food. So instead of wasting several hours each day cooking, baking and preparing unhealthy foods, we have more time to do more important things.

If we take the example of a student who has to work a paid job to help fund his studies, he or she doesn't have time to cook and prepare food so has two choices;

#1. The student has to eat fast food to save time which will undoubtedly affect his or her health in the long term.

#2. The student can go raw and eat natural foods as much as possible thus saving time, money and benefiting his or her health.

When it comes to attending certain ceremonies, vegans and raw vegans maybe face some difficulties. This is because we live in a society where meat and unhealthy foods are very popular at such events, even more popular than natural foods. I see this as a way of correcting certain traditions in society as there are many different creative ways to present natural food for ceremonies and big party events. Many talented vegan and raw vegan chefs have created tasty and healthy recipes which can inspire us to do the same. By providing such foods at these events, you can help change the perception of natural food.

Equally for a vegan guest, a shared meal is an occasion to inform others about their healthy diet.

Friendship, cordiality, and good social relations don't conflict with veganism. Food is only one aspect of a celebration, so it is not logical for a vegan or raw food eater to shy away from their true manner. Hence, it is possible to remain vegan or a raw food eater in almost every situation, even at parties and with friends who are not vegan. It's better to inform all friends of this pure and true-hearted lifestyle.

Some people think that veganism/raw foodism is a radical manner or a strict religion, but really, it is just a simple lifestyle based on a natural human need. However some vegan individuals may become fanatical, but the truth is that peace is the basic philosophy of this lifestyle.

Veganism and Morality

Morality means different things to different people. It doesn't have a special and unique definition. The meaning of morality can be flexible depending on situations because it's a mental and thinking subject so our definition of it is dynamic, not static.

Bearing this is mind I would like to explore why humans think it is acceptable to deprive some animals of life. With the increasing popularity of plant-based diets there isn't a lack of food which is forcing us to kill innocent animals for our bellies. But still humans incarcerate animals and torture them with hormones and drugs.

When we use our mind, we understand that animals are not created by God or nature to be tortured and killed by humans for food. Maybe there is at least one reason for creating them and it wasn't to feed humans. If you look a little deeper, you will see that all creatures stabilize equivalency in different cycles of nature. Nothing is perfect so all creatures go forward to perfection together by helping each other.

On the basis of natural laws, plants are the main factor of each food continuum which life is impossible without. Herbivores have a very important role in nature and the ecosystem. According to the article *'Plants Can Benefit from Herbivory'* from Plos One[189]:

"Plants and herbivores can evolve beneficial interactions. Growth factors found in animal saliva are probably key factors underlying plant compensatory responses to herbivory. However, there is still a lack of knowledge about how animal saliva interacts with herbivory intensities and how saliva can mobilize photosynthate reserves in damaged plants."

In the article: *'Large herbivores can play critical role in maintaining ecosystem health'*, scientists from Stanford University, Princeton University and the University of California-Davis, carried out a study where large herbivorous mammals were excluded from experimental plots to monitor changes to the ecosystem[190]. The study concluded:

"While top predators are undeniably important to ecological function, this new study shows that large herbivores can also play critical roles."

Different animals have made different positive contributions to our environment, depending on their own physical system and instincts. There are different theories about the coming into existence of carnivorous animals, but it's not logical to presume that because carnivores live on earth, there is no problem if humans eat meat, too. There are so many differences between animals and us, including body type. Also it is apparent that no wild animal in nature keeps other animals caged so they will become fat and then kills and burns them before they can be consumed. Wild animals kill their bait in just a few seconds without causing any long-term suffering.

A very shameful example of animal cruelty is foie gras (pronounced "fwah grah") which is French for fatty liver. It is an expensive appetizer produced by force-feeding ducks or geese two or three times daily through a pipe shoved down their throats. The force-feeding can cause painful bruising, lacerations, sores, and tearing of the birds' throats. Due to this unhealthy and unnatural diet, the birds' livers can swell up to ten times their normal size and become sick, a medical condition called hepatic lipidosis, and cease to function properly. This harrowing process and its effects on the birds make it difficult for them to walk or even breathe comfortably. The birds are then slaughtered at just three months old and many die before they reach that age.

Many humane and animal rights organizations are working to prevent force-feeding birds to make foie gras. These efforts are supported by veterinarians, ethicists, religious, political, and business leaders, including restaurant chefs and farmers. You can find more information about it on the No Foie Gras campaign website: http://www.NoFoieGras.org [191]

there are two pictures in the next page related to Foie Gras :

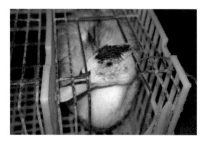

They suffer from stomach ache and foot edema

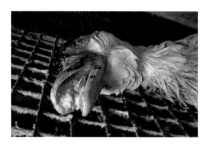

This bird died from force-feeding

Before eating, we should think about what we eat and pay attention to our health and the life of animals. A food which is produced by torturing animals will not give us anything except toxins, cancer and other diseases.

There are some people, like the French philosopher René Descartes, who believed that animals don't have souls and don't feel pain and there are other people who believe that animals have sprit, intellect and personality like humans so it's necessary to observe their rights.

Many scientific experiments have proved that meat and animal products are harmful for our bodies[192], while fruit and vegetables are vital for our bodies because of our body anatomy. If we think wisely, we will understand there is no reason to kill animals for food and that there are various delicious plants which will supply all of our nutritional needs.

Wild animals kill other animals only when they are hungry and because of their inability to obtain their needs from plants. But humans have access to all kinds of food and cultivate their own. Unfortunately many of us rear animals in barbaric conditions and then kill them so they can produce different kinds of unnatural foods like sausages, frankfurters, barbecued and conserved foods while often adding more toxins to preserve or make them more tasty. It's amazing that anyone expects to remain healthy after eating such junk food.

The social advantage of becoming a vegetarian and respecting animal rights is explored in the book '*Animal Rights as a Post Citizenship Movement*' by Brian Lowe and Caryn Ginsberg.[193]

Nowadays it has been proven that at the very least vertebrates feel pain because they have a central nervous system. Those that have studied animals and dedicated their work to researching creatures have also reported how animals experience many different feelings. Animals enjoy sexual relations, love their babies and sometimes love the babies of other species, proving they have sagacity.

The belief, such as that of Descartes, that animals are like apathetic robots or machines, is invalid today because we know more about animals. The idea that we would engage in bullfighting or sacrifice animals like some tribes do for religious or traditional rituals, is not logical at all; it's completely futile and delusive.

We know that some animals which are factory farmed become sick and their lifespan is shortened due to the cruelties they have to endure so they cannot be healthy food for humans.

If a wild animal attacks a human, the human will do everything it can to defend itself. It therefore makes no sense that humans hurt and kill those animals which don't hurt humans and their meat isn't suitable and necessary for us to eat, while fruits and plant foods exist in abundance.

The honey debate

Some view honey as an herbal food and others recognize that it's a food that has come from a living creature. But when deciding whether we should or should not eat honey, two aspects of this debate should be taken into consideration: First, the nutritional view and second, the ethical view.

To consider the nutritional aspect, one of the incomparable features of honey is that it never putrefies at all. Honey is antibacterial so has some benefits and it seems that using it occasionally (and not every day) is not harmful for the body.

There are some natural toxins in honey, the natural toxins which exist in flowers and also those toxins which are later added by the bees[194]. Honey is also slightly acidic and prolonged exposure to acidic foods can erode tooth enamel and the linings of your esophagus, stomach and intestines, which can lead to acid reflux disease.

Eating too much honey (more than 10 tbsp. daily) causes gastric problems such as stomach cramps, bloating and diarrhea. Due to honey's fructose content, eating too much also might interfere with the small intestine's ability to absorb nutrients. This can contribute to further abdominal discomfort until the honey is out of your system.

Honey is too much for an infant as some honey contains botulism spores, which the immature digestive system of an infant cannot handle, leading to botulism poisoning. The signs of botulism are constipation, weakness, listlessness and decreased appetite. Uncontrolled botulism causes muscle paralysis and eventually death. Because of this risk, pediatricians recommend no honey for children under 12 months or for pregnant or breastfeeding women. Botulism can be treated if detected early and usually leads to a full recovery.[195]

Considering the nutritional aspect I would conclude that honey could be a medicine but it's not a complete food. We cannot eat a meal only of honey as we could of fruit.

To turn to the ethical aspect of eating honey, there are some beekeepers who feed honeybees refined sugar or non-natural syrup, which can harm the bees' system, such as weakening their defense[196], and has negative effects on the quality of the honey as artificially produced sugar and syrup is not a natural food for bees.[197]

This act is carried out so more money can be made but to presume that we have the right to carry out such an act is foolish.

If anyone thinks animal rights are not meaningful for these creatures because they are insects and very small, he/she is mistaken.

Yes, the honeybee is tiny yet the life of humans and other animals depends on the endeavors of this small and beautiful creature, because it increases the efficiency of herbal products with its pollination performance.

Bees may produce more honey than they need, but why should we think they produce this extra honey for our consumption? The output of herbal productions would be greatly decreased and all land creatures would become extinct without the pollination action of honeybees. These creatures have a desire to live like any other creature so they produce more honey than they need in order to have extra food during winter or in the case of drought, they can use this extra honey to survive until conditions change.[198]

As some mountaineers have reported bees sometimes leave the extra honey in the old hive, seal the entrance with bees wax and continue their pollination. It seems they don't need that honey. In cases of emergencies perhaps it can be of help to other bees for example if bees in other hives run out of food during winter or in a drought and there is no pollen for them, maybe they can use the extra honey from a hive in another place for survival.

Thus, the honeybee is a very important and useful creature for all other living beings on earth. But they produce honey for their own use, and although a bear who finds an abandoned hive can use its honey, if bees see it, they will sting the bear. According to a Persian book called the *'Language of Foods'*,[199] in some desert parts of Iran, honey from local bees is toxic for humans, because those bees are exposed to very toxic herbs, so their honey is also toxic for other animals. The interesting point is that honeybees are important even in deserts. It seems they are not supposed to produce honey for human consumption, but their pollination never stops even in harsh desert lands.

Vegans have many different reasons as to why they don't eat honey such as the killing of bees due to bad keeping and moving beehives, the fact that some bees are forced to produce more honey because humans take their honey, like the way hens are forced to lay more eggs[200] or cows are forced to produce more milk[201]. These are maybe indicators that some hormonal changes have happened in their body because of compulsive conditions which can't be counted as very natural. Honeybees are very sensitive, so much so that they may suffer due to mobile phone radiation[202].

Pure natural honey is very scarce and very expensive and the human population has grown so much that it's impossible to have natural honey for everyone so we should find alternatives. Sweet fruit such as grapes and date palms along with their molasses is much cheaper than honey and contain many antioxidants, anti-bacterial compounds, minerals and anti-cancer properties. Certainly, each useful thing which exists in honey also exists in herbs and plants, because honeybees get them from different herbs, so we can supply all the useful content of honey, so no animal product is necessary for humans.

My recommendation is to gradually reduce your honey intake if it's not possible to cut it out completely. We don't need to eat honey every day. Instead, with the help of honeybees in vegan and organic gardening, we can utilize them in a completely moral and eco-friendly manner by their pollination which creates more products of better quality, while letting them enjoy their efforts by leaving them alone and not using their honey.

Morality isn't a limited thing; it needs to be thought about very much and if you do so well, you will find that there is no justification for torturing animals. It's more important that we teach these lessons to the next generation and the children of the future because they expect a better world, as much as we do.

A spotlight on vegetarianism

Many famous people have become vegetarian during their life for the sake of remaining healthy, observing animal rights, or both. Great men and women like: Buddha, Zartosht (Iranian Prophet), Leo Tolstoy (famous Russian author), George Bernard-Shaw, Charles Darwin, Gandhi, Newton, Leonardo Da Vinci, Albert Einstein, Ralph Waldo Emerson, Sergey Brin (Co-founder of Google), Joe Namath (football player), Robert Cheeke (vegan bodybuilder), Scott Jurek (the multiple winner of 100-mile races and twice winner of the Badwater Ultra Marathon)203 and many scientists, philosophers, actors and athletes are vegetarian.[204] Although most of them aren't vegan I would like to use some quotes from these people on the subject of animal rights, health and eating meat:

"The world, we are told, was made especially for man – a presumption not supported by all the facts.... Why should man value himself as more than a small part of the one great unit of creation?"
~ JOHN MUIR, NATURALIST AND EXPLORER (1838–1914)

"There is no fundamental difference between man and the higher animals in their mental faculties.... The lower animals, like man, manifestly feel pleasure and pain, happiness, and misery."
"The love for all living creatures is the most noble attribute of man."
~ Charles Darwin, naturalist and author (1809–1882)

"Even in the worm that crawls in the earth there glows a divine spark. When you slaughter a creature, you slaughter God."
"As long as people will shed the blood of innocent creatures there can be no peace, no liberty, no harmony between people. Slaughter and justice cannot dwell together."
"When a human being kills an animal for food, he is neglecting his own hunger for justice. Man prays for mercy, but is unwilling to extend it to others. Why then should man expect mercy from God? It is unfair to expect something that you are not willing to give."
~ ISAAC BASHEVIS SINGER, WRITER AND NOBEL LAUREATE

"I don't hold animals superior or even equal to humans. The whole case for behaving decently to animals rests on the fact that we are the superior species. We are the species uniquely capable of imagination, rationality, and moral choice – and that is precisely why we are under an obligation to recognize and respect the rights of animals."
~ *BRIGID BROPHY (1929–1995)*

"If you visit the killing floor of a slaughterhouse, it will brand your soul for life."
~ *HOWARD LYMAN, AUTHOR OF* Mad Cowboy

"In fact, if one person is unkind to an animal it is considered to be cruelty, but where a lot of people are unkind to animals, especially in the name of commerce, the cruelty is condoned and, once large sums of money are at stake, will be defended to the last by otherwise intelligent people."
~ *RUTH HARRISON, AUTHOR OF* Animal Machines

"It is a sobering thought that animals could do without man, yet man would find it almost impossible to do without animals."
~ *RUTH HARRISON*

"Now I can look at you in peace; I don't eat you anymore."
~ *FRANZ KAFKA, WHILE ADMIRING FISH IN AN AQUARIUM*

"The beef industry has contributed to more American deaths than all the wars of this century, all natural disasters, and all automobile accidents combined. If beef is your idea of "real food for real people," you'd better live real close to a real good hospital."
~ *NEAL D. BARNARD, MD, PRESIDENT, PHYSICIANS COMMITTEE FOR RESPONSIBLE MEDICINE*

"I have been following a vegan diet now since the 1980s, and find it not only healthier, but also much more attractive than the chunks of meat that were on my plate as a child."
~ *NEAL D. BARNARD*

"Can you really ask what reason Pythagoras had for abstaining from flesh? For my part I rather wonder both by what accident and in what state of soul or mind the first man did so, touched his mouth to gore and brought his lips to the flesh of a dead creature, he who set forth tables of dead, stale bodies and ventured to call food and nourishment the parts that had a little before bellowed and cried, moved and lived. How could his eyes endure the slaughter when throats were slit and hides flayed and limbs torn from limb? How could his nose endure the stench? How was it that the pollution did not turn away his taste, which made contact with the sores of others and sucked juices and serums from mortal wounds?... It is certainly not lions and wolves that we eat out of self-defense; on the contrary, we ignore these and slaughter harmless, tame creatures without stings or teeth to harm us, creatures that, I swear, nature appears to have produced for the sake of their beauty and grace. But nothing abashed us, not the flower-like tinting of the flesh, not the persuasiveness of the harmonious voice, not the cleanliness of their habits or the unusual intelligence that may be found in the poor wretches. No, for the sake of a little flesh we deprive them of sun, of light, of the duration of life to which they are entitled by birth and being."
~ Plutarch

"When a man wants to murder a tiger, he calls it sport; when a tiger wants to murder him, he calls it ferocity."
"Animals are my friends, and I don't eat my friends."
"A man of my spiritual intensity does not eat corpses."
"Think of the fierce energy concentrated in an acorn! You bury it in the ground, and it explodes into an oak! Bury a sheep, and nothing happens but decay."
~ George Bernard Shaw, writer and Nobel laureate (1856–1950)

"It is my view that the vegetarian manner of living, by its purely physical effect on the human temperament, would most beneficially influence the lot of mankind."

"A human being is a part of the whole, called by us the "Universe," a part limited in time and space. He experiences himself, his thoughts and feelings, as something separate from the rest – a kind of optical delusion of his consciousness. This delusion is a kind of prison for us, restricting us to our personal desires and to affection for a few persons nearest to us. Our task must be to free ourselves from this prison by widening our circle of compassion to embrace all living creatures and the whole of nature in its beauty. Nobody is able to achieve this completely, but the striving for such achievement is in itself a part of the liberation and a foundation for inner security."

"If a man aspires towards a righteous life, his first act of abstinence is from injury to animals,"

"Nothing will benefit human health and increase chances for survival of life on Earth as much as the evolution to a vegetarian diet."
~Albert Einstein

"As long as men massacre animals, they will kill each other. Indeed, he who sows the seeds of murder and pain cannot reap the joy of love."
~ Pythagoras

"Non-violence leads to the highest ethics, which is the goal of all evolution. Until we stop harming all other living beings, we are still savages."

"The doctor of the future will give no medicine, but will instruct his patient in the care of the human frame, in diet and in the cause and prevention of disease."
~ Thomas Edison, American inventor and Businessman

"A dead cow or sheep lying in the pasture is recognized as carrion. The same sort of carcass dressed and hung up in a butcher's stall passes as food."
~ John Harvey Kellogg, American physician (1852–1943)

"For me, going vegan was an ethical and environmental decision. I'm doing the right thing by the animals."

"My respect and empathy towards animals includes sea dwellers too - from dolphins to fish to lobsters. So, of course, I wouldn't dream of eating them."

~ Alexandra Paul, Actress

"How can you eat anything with eyes?"
~Will Kellogg

"I grew up in cattle country--that's why I became a vegetarian. Meat stinks, for the animals, the environment, and your health."
"We all love animals. Why do we call some "pets" and others "dinner?""
~K. D. Lang

"As custodians of the planet it is our responsibility to deal with all species with kindness, love and compassion. That these animals suffer through human cruelty is beyond understanding. Please help to stop this madness."
"People get offended by animal rights campaigns. It's ludicrous. It's not as bad as mass animal death in a factory."
~ Richard Gere

"Compassion is the foundation of everything positive, everything good. If you carry the power of compassion to the marketplace and the dinner table, you can make your life really count."
~ Rue McClanahan

"Thousands of animals [now millions] are butchered every day without a shadow of remorse. It cries vengeance upon all the human race."
~Romain Rolland

"I have since an early age abjured the use of meat, and the time will come when men such as I will look upon the murder of animals as they now look upon the murder of men."
~ Leonardo Da Vinci

"Until he extends the circle of his compassion to all living things, man will not himself find peace."
~ Albert Schweitzer, philosopher, physician, and musician (Nobel 1952)

"Wild animals never kill for sport. Man is the only one to whom the torture and death of his fellow creatures is amusing in itself."
~ James A. Froude, English historian (1818–1894)

"You have just dined, and however scrupulously the slaughterhouse is concealed in the graceful distance of miles, there is complicity."
~Ralph Waldo Emerson

" "Thou shall not kill" does not apply to murder of one's own kind only, but to all living beings; and this Commandment was inscribed in the human breast long before it was proclaimed from Sinai."
"If a man earnestly seeks a righteous life, his first act of abstinence is from animal food."
"If he be really and seriously seeking to live a good life, the first thing from which he will abstain will always be the use of animal food, because ...its use is simply immoral, as it involves the performance of an act which is contrary to the moral feeling: killing!"
~Leo Tolstoy

"I think if you want to eat more meat you should kill it yourself and eat it raw so that you are not blinded by the hypocrisy of having it processed for you."
~Margi Clark

"Recognize meat for what it really is: the antibiotic- and pesticide-laden corpse of a tortured animal."
~Ingrid Newkirk

"Cruelty to animals can become violence to humans."
~ Ali MacGraw

"If slaughterhouses had glass walls, everyone would be a vegetarian."
~Paul McCartney

"For hundreds of thousands of years the stew in the pot has brewed hatred and resentment that is difficult to stop. If you wish to know why there are disasters of armies and weapons in the world, just listen to the piteous cries from the slaughterhouse in the midnight."

~Poem by a Chinese monk

"About 2,000 pounds of grains must be supplied to livestock in order to produce enough meat and other livestock products to support a person for a year, whereas 400 pounds of grain eaten directly will support a person for a year. Thus, a given quantity of grain eaten directly will feed 5 times as many people as it will if it is eaten indirectly by humans in the form of livestock products…"
~M.E. ENSMINGER, PHD

"May all that have life be delivered from suffering."
~Buddha

"Martin Luther King taught us all nonviolence. I was told to extend nonviolence to the mother and her calf."
~Dick Gregory

"Once I was fishing and caught the hook in the fish's eye. That was the last time I ate a killed creature."
~ Janet Barkas, editor of Grove Press

"Many things made me become a vegetarian, among them the higher food yield as a solution to world hunger."
~ John Denver

"Since visiting the abattoirs [slaughterhouses] of South France, I have stopped eating meat."
~ Vincent Van Gogh

"I spoke often in Congress against the war in Vietnam and commented on Congresspersons hiding from the reality of war by saying, "Many eat the meat, but few go to the slaughterhouse". I said it so often I became a vegetarian."
~ Rep. Andrew Jacobs, formerly of Indianapolis

"The other members of the National Football League say I'm in the minority ... but they are. A majority of the world is vegetarian."
~ Former Pittsburgh Steeler and New York Giant football player Glenn Scolnick

"I have no doubt that it is a part of the destiny of the human race, in its gradual improvement, to leave off eating animals, as surely as the savage tribes have left off eating each other..."
~ Henry David Thoreau

"If [man] is not to stifle his human feelings, he must practice kindness towards animals, for he who is cruel to animals becomes hard also in his dealings with men. We can judge the heart of a man by his treatment of animals."
~ Immanuel Kant

"Humans are the only hunters who kill when not hungry."
~ Steven Spielberg

"It is a surprisingly close progression from hunting animals to hunting and torturing people... catching and lynching blacks or smoking out Jews during the Holocaust."
~ Aviva Cantor writing in Ms. Magazine

"Arson and cruelty to animals are two of three childhood warning signs regarding the potential to be a serial killer."
~ John Douglas, profiler of serial killers for the FBI, upon whom the FBI character in "Silence of the Lambs" was based

"You put a baby in a crib with an apple and a rabbit. If it eats the rabbit and plays with the apple, I'll buy you a new car!"
~Harvey Diamond

"To my mind, the life of a lamb is no less precious than that of a human being. I should be unwilling to take the life of a lamb for the sake of the human body."
"The greatness of a nation and its moral progress can be judged by the way its animals are treated... I hold that, the more helpless a creature, the more entitled it is to protection by man from the cruelty of man."
~ Mahatma Gandhi

"I will not eat anything that walks, runs, skips, hops or crawls. God knows that I've crawled on occasion, and I'm glad that no one ate me."
~Alex Poulos

"People often say that humans have always eaten animals, as if this is a justification for continuing the practice. According to this logic, we should not try to prevent people from murdering other people, since this has also been done since the earliest of times!"
~ Isaac Singer

"Thanksgiving dinner's sad and thankless
Christmas dinner's dark and blue
When you stop and try to see it
From the turkey's point of view."
~Shel Silverstein, "Point of View"

"It is difficult to picture the great Creator conceiving of a program of one creature (which he has made) using another living creature for purposes of experimentation. There must be other, less cruel ways of obtaining knowledge."
~ ADLAI STEVENSON, AMERICAN STATESMAN (1835–1914)

"We must educate the public. The average person has no idea of what's going on in factory farms, in laboratories, circuses, roadside zoos or rodeos."
~ Bob Barker

"Do we, as humans, having an ability to reason and to communicate abstract ideas verbally and in writing, and to form ethical and moral judgments using the accumulated knowledge of the ages, have the right to take the lives of other sentient organisms, particularly when we are not forced to do so by hunger or dietary need, but rather do so for the somewhat frivolous reason that we like the taste of meat?"
~ Peter Cheeke (PhD, Contemporary issues in Animal Agriculture 2004 textbook)

"If any kid ever realized what was involved in factory farming they would never touch meat again. I was so moved by the intelligence, sense of fun and personalities of the animals I worked with on Babe that by the end of the film I was a vegetarian."
~ James Cromwell

"Feeding plants to animals then eating the animals is like filtering water through a sewer then drinking it!"
~ Bruce Friedrich

"The highest realms of thought are impossible to reach without first attaining an understanding of compassion."
~ Socrates

"The first time I ever entered a battery house (chicken farm), I thought it was the entrance to Hell."
~ Violet Spalding

"We consume the carcasses of creatures of like appetites, passions and organs with our own, and fill the slaughterhouses daily with screams of fear and pain."
~ Robert Louis Stevenson

"Your...life may be of no consequence to anyone else but is invaluable to you because it's the only one you've got. Exactly the same is true of each individual deer, hare, rabbit, fox, fish, pheasant and butterfly." ~ Unknown

"The animals of the world exist for their own reasons. They were not made for humans any more than black people were made for whites or women for men."
~ Alice Walker

And please remember this general one:

"You are not required to complete the task of repairing the world, neither are you free to abstain from it." ~ **Pirke Avot**

Conclusion

There are many resources in nature which can be useful or harmful depending on how we use them. For example, oil, gas and coal are natural resources from which we can produce many different things, but unfortunately 80% of them are burnt in cars and factories, making our air more polluted.

If solar energy, eco-friendly cars and other green energy solutions become popular, these natural fossil resources can be used for producing instead of burning, which will greatly improve our environment. However, the first and most important step still is to change ourselves and improve our diet. Without it, other steps cannot be done completely.

To quote from the book '*Advantages of Vegetarianism*' by the Iranian author and novelist Sadegh Hedayat:

"If generations of humans should reach the top of development and perfection, it will be in a natural environment with plant foods, because meat-eating and factitive civilization has depraved him and taken him away to extirpation, unless a new and fecund generation of humans whose life is compatible with natural laws, become inherited instead of him, if not, his generation will disappear in a disgraceful manner."

Each human harms the environment directly or indirectly during his lifetime, for example engaging in fishing as a calming recreational activity, yet is going against nature rather than being part of it. Gardening is a pleasurable hobby which provides good and positive feelings when we see the fruits of our labor grow and produce crops or beautiful flowers. There are better alternatives instead of unworthy cruel activities which damage nature. So follow a positive manner to get satisfying results both for you and your environment.

I hope that everyone can do something useful for the world to secure our beautiful surroundings for future generations.

As we enter a new age, change is certainly necessary. But we should also be careful to choose the best changes that we can. Thus, we can be hopeful that we experience the most blissful and happy life on this planet.

References

Here are the books and websites which I have referred to, with the authors' permission. They are good resources for anyone who wants to do more research:

The 80/10/10 Diet – Balancing Your Health, Your Weight, and Your Life One Luscious Bite at a Time_ Dr. Douglas N. Graham_ 2006

*Raw Secrets_* by Frederic Patenaude

The website of Gholam Hossein Khorsand, an Iranian nutrition researcher: *www.Khorsand.org*

Persian books on a natural diet by Nosratollah Javid_ 2012-2013 (not available in other languages as of 2015) entitled The Secrets of Natural Foods and The Secrets of Natural Treatment

Official website of Iran Vegetarian Society: *http://www.iranvegetarians.com*

Official website of Dr. Zarin Azar: *www.zarinazar.com*

Live-Eating (raw-eating), Philosophy of Feeding Health_ by Arshavir Ter-Hovanessian (Persian Version), 4th edition, 1976, Tehran

Cooked-Eating, a Lethal Addiction_ by Arshavir Ter-Hovanessian, 1976

Raw-eating; both food and treatment (Persian)_ by Ali Akbar RadPooya_7[th] edition, 1997

Advantages of Vegetarianism (Persian)_ by Sadegh Hedayat_ 1927

Dr. Abdolhossein Navab's books written in Persian entitled Raw Veganism and Using Natural Rules in a Healthy Life.

Language of Foods (Persian Version), by Dr. Ghiassedin Jazayeri

Natural Cures "They" Don't Want You to know about, by Kevin Trudeau, 2004

Life Without Cancer: How to Stop Making Disease in Your Body, by Andrea Lambert, 2013

Dr T. Colin Campbell's website: *http://www.tcolincampbell.org/*

The valuable experiences of Mango_ a vegetarian from his youth and an experienced raw vegan now:
http://MangoDurian.blogspot.com and *www.fruitnut.net*

About the Author

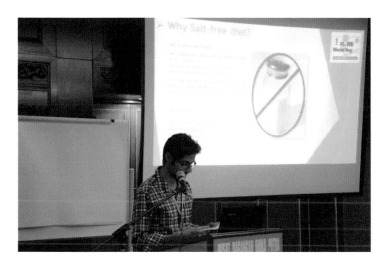

I am a 21-year-old student of life. I was born in Iran (Persia), a beautiful country, but at the same time, a country full of troubles. All countries are beautiful and have their own troubles, but I think there is something about the troubles Iran has that are different; you have to experience them by living in country under global boycott to understand what I'm saying.

The most important thing that I can tell you about myself is that I was always a very curious boy, curious about everything. My curiosity helped me a lot, but sometimes it produced difficulties; yet without curiosity, mankind would become a robot, or a zombie.

I'm a blogger and started blogging in 2007 (of course in Persian). I still believe that I'm not a professional blogger yet, but I enjoy it very much when I record my thoughts. I read many blogs (in Persian and English), which I find a fun way to learn new things and stay updated.

I became a raw vegan after suffering severe headaches and some digestive disorders for several years, and as I witnessed sicknesses in others, I thought that maybe this was not a natural phenomenon to get sick. Surely there was a way to cure and prevent many sicknesses. So I started to do some research in my free time, by reading books, magazines, newspapers, and of course, online.

As chemical medical drugs have negative side effects, I always avoided them as much as possible and instead, I tried natural therapies to prevent and cure diseases. I was also very interested in natural therapies and started to research this subject.

I became a vegan in October 2011. I spent more time researching nutrition, read more books and articles (both in Persian and English), and wrote my own e-book in Persian about living the vegan lifestyle. I have edited my Persian e-book four times and published it successfully on Persian websites.

I also have my own Persian and English websites, and I am in contact with many vegetarians in Iran and other countries, talking to them about their experiences so I can learn more about the vegan lifestyle.

As there were very limited Persian resources about vegetarianism when I started, my friends and I wanted to help the Persian community access more information (including free e-books and documentary videos) easily, and that's our honor to help Iranian people know more about natural-based lifestyles like other nations do.

But I really do not limit this information to my nationality. So I decided to continue my activities globally, and maybe I can help more people all over the world, which is a holy purpose for me.

I started to translate my book from Persian to English, as I passed the ESL (English as Second Language) courses, and it was becoming vital for me to spread the message. So I continued my research and during this time I edited both the Persian and English versions of my books and completed them.

However, my English book had some foreign readers, and they told me that I needed to get help from a professional editor, and they were right. So I took it to Louise Scrivens, and I'm thankful for her endeavors.

Now I have different ideas for both my websites and I'm looking for good partners to produce useful articles. Here is the address of my English website:

www.VeganIdealWorld.com

And this is my Persian website, which at the time this was written, has the largest Persian vegetarian file, including e-books, documentary movies, and clips related to vegetarianism and natural health:

www.VeganDownload.com

To provide a better service, I decided to set up a separate website for this book so it makes it easier to record news about this book and readers' feedback and experiences:

www.RethinkYourDiet.com

You are welcome to share your ideas, experiences and suggestions with me via the contact form, email, or Facebook.

In 2013, I searched the web to find out about vegetarian festivals around the world and discovered the 41st International Vegetarian Festival due to take place in Malaysia in October of that year. I contacted the Vegetarian Society of Malaysia via email and introduced myself, submitted my book and resume and enrolled in their speaking program. After two months, they kindly accepted me as a speaker at the festival, and I was so happy to be given the chance to speak about what I love. (The picture above is me speaking at the festival).

At the festival I spoke about fruit-based and salt-free raw vegan diets; a subject which is not accepted by all experts. But I was still happy and satisfied to speak about what I believe is true, supported with scientific reasons and personal experiences.

I've uploaded my speech and slide shows, which I presented at the vegetarian festival. If you want to download it and have a look, you can contact me via email at:

Moin.Ghn@gmail.com

Life has many ups and downs, and I have faced many difficulties so far both within my family and financially. Thankfully I have gotten through them, but I still face many challenges such as continuing my academic education, as it was not possible for me to go to university after gaining my high school diploma.

I've learned many lessons in life, and am thankful for that. I think spirituality is not limited to one special religion; it's a powerful tendency inside human beings which is about finding harmony. Life will become joyful and meaningful with love, especially unconditional love.

I'm interested in many fields, and I think we need to nurture our abilities, do something useful, and even invent something new. With creativity we can realize our hidden potential and know ourselves better.

I don't categorize myself, and I try to avoid the term "-ism" because I think we should see the facts without any prejudging. So in this book, I have tried to explain what I've learned during this time about nutrition without any fanaticism. Please remember that when we use the word "veganism" it just refers to a lifestyle and its purpose. The word "veganism" is not very important because a vegan/raw vegan believes his behavior is natural, so there is nothing to categorize as different.

Unconscious following is just a waste of time and energy as we are here to experience a conscious life. So if we choose our manner consciously, we won't have many difficulties in life. Conscious power will help us to live in the best possible state.

I hope that all of us become healthy, happy and blissful.

Your sincere brother,
Moein Ghahremani Nejad

All footnotes/references of this book

Below are all the references/footnotes/endnotes in this book .I had to convert all footnotes in this book to end notes, as it was necessary to publish book in a format which would be usable by all devices .

---

[1] Khan Academy is a non-profit educational website created in 2006. More information can be found online.

[2] The following section has been translated from Persian to English by Ali Asghar JannatPour and edited by myself.

[3] The following extract from Mr. Khorsand's diaries and story has been translated from Persian to English by Javid Shadi and edited by myself.

[4] Read the complete article 'Enzymes: Are They for Real?':
http://foodnsport.com/blog/Enzymes-Are-They-for-Real.html

Also watch the video ' Raw Food Enzyme Myth Exposed by Dr. Graham' on Youtube:
http://www.youtube.com/watch?v=V951nGyKIYM

[5] *'The Cold Truth About Raw Food Diets'* by Dr. Joel Fuhrman:
http://www.diseaseproof.com/archives/healthy-food-the-cold-truth-about-raw-food-diets.html

[6] For more information, read the article *'Elephants Eat Dirt to Supplement Sodium'* :
http://scienceblog.com/983/elephants-eat-dirt-to-supplement-sodium

[7] For more information, refer to the article ' *Eat Dirt*: In the competition between parrots and fruit trees, it's the winners who bite the dust.': *http://discovermagazine.com/1998/feb/eatdirt1408*

[8] ' Oxygenate your body - How to restore oxygen balance and help prevent disease':
http://www.naturalnews.com/032096_oxygenation_body.html

The QR codes related to 6-9 in Sequence (from left):

[9] The explanations are adopted from different sources, including:
PETA (People for the Ethical Treatment of Animals): www.PETA.org
PCRM (Physicians Committee for Responsible medicine): www.PCRM.org
www.EarthSave.ca
Pages 16-18 of the book *'The 80/10/10 Diet:* Balancing your health, your weight, and your life One Luscious Bite at a Time' by Dr. Douglas N. Graham_ 2006

[10] You can read more about this in various books such as: *'What's Wrong with Eating Meat?'* by Barbara Parham, 1979

[11] For more information, refer to *'the China Study'* book by Dr. T. Colin Campbell.

The website of Dr T. Colin Campbell: *http://www.tcolincampbell.org/*

and his academic page on the website of Cornell University:
http://www.human.cornell.edu/bio.cfm?netid=tcc1

The QR codes related to links above Sequence at next page(from left):

[12] *http://www.earthsave.ca/files/anatomy.pdf*

[13] PDF Version of the mentioned paper: *http://www.earthsave.ca/files/anatomy.pdf*

[14] A well-known Canadian Raw Foodist

[15] He is a natural hygienist. Here is an English version of interview with Albert Mosséri on Frederic Patenaude's website: *http://www.fredericpatenaude.com/articles/interview-mosseri.html*

[16] Dean Karnazes is an American ultramarathon runner, and author of Ultramarathon Man

[17] See the article '*Born to Run*' from the May 2006 issue: *http://discovermagazine.com/2006/may/tramps-like-us*

[18] See the article: '*How Long can a person survive without food?*' in Scientific American: *http://www.scientificamerican.com/article/how-long-can-a-person-sur/*

[19] The info graphic in LiveScience about Americans: *http://www.livescience.com/18070-food-americans-eat-year-infographic.html*

The QR codes related to 15, 17, 18 and 19 in sequence (from left):

[20] Watch the video '*100% Raw Vegan Day 10 True Hunger vs. False Hunger*': *https://www.youtube.com/watch?v=Hmeu4Jj3wQM*

[21] Read the article '*True hunger vs. False hunger*' by Mike Dillman: *http://www.realworldraw.com/raw-blog/2010/5/25/true-hunger-vs-false-hunger.html*

[22] See the article on National Geographic: '*How do Giant Pandas Survive on Bamboo Diets?*': *http://news.nationalgeographic.com/news/2011/10/111017-pandas-bamboo-bacteria-plants-meat-bears-animals-science/*

[23] Read the article '*When Big Carnivores Go Down, Even Vegetarians Take The Hit*' on National public radio: *http://www.npr.org/2014/01/10/261120968/when-big-carnivores-go-down-even-vegetarians-take-the-hit*

The QR codes related to 20-23 in sequence (from left):

[24] Search in the Internet for complete report, for example here are two sources: *http://io9.com/5911739/worlds-first-vegetarian-shark-spurns-meat-for-celery-sticks* *http://www.treehugger.com/natural-sciences/worlds-first-vegetarian-shark-prefers-lettuce.html*

[25] 'Earliest ancestor of land herbivores discovered: 300-million-year-old predator showed way to modern terrestrial ecosystem': *http://www.sciencedaily.com/releases/2014/04/140416172243.htm*

'Evolutionary history of what mammals eat: Some groups of mammals have changed their feeding strategies over time': *http://www.sciencedaily.com/releases/2012/04/120416154417.htm*

The QR codes related to 24-25 in sequence (from left):

[26] Read the article '*Are Dogs Carnivores — or Omnivores?*':
http://www.dogfoodadvisor.com/canine-nutrition/dogs-carnivores-omnivores/

[27] Read the articles:
'*Should Your Pet Go on a Vegetarian Diet?*': http://pets.webmd.com/features/vegetarian-diet-dogs-cats

'*Is a vegetarian diet safe for my dog?*': *http://www.mnn.com/earth-matters/animals/stories/is-a-vegetarian-diet-safe-for-my-dog*

[28] Some more resources related to vegetarian/vegan diet and health:
E Pinhey, J Ortiz: '*Health Advantages of a Vegetarian Diet*' _ Available here for download:
http://dana.ucc.nau.edu/ejp32/Argumentative.doc

'57 Health Benefits of Going Vegan': http://www.nursingdegree.net/blog/19/57-health-benefits-of-going-vegan/

'What Is A Vegan Diet? What Are The Benefits Of Being Vegan?':
http://www.medicalnewstoday.com/articles/149636.php

'*Health, ethics and environment: A qualitative study of vegetarian motivations*'_ by Nick Fox, Katie Ward_ School of Health and Related Research, University of Sheffield, UK:
http://www.sciencedirect.com/science/article/pii/S0195666307003686

The QR codes related to links above, in sequence in next page (from left):

[29] All FAQs of Dr. Zarin Azar in Persian are available on her website: *www.ZarinAzar.com*

[30] Cancer cells can by fed by the sugar in any type of food, as they can eat more sugar than regular cells. For more information:

'Mechanism that makes tumor cells sugar addicted discovered': *http://www.sciencedaily.com/releases/2014/04/140404092937.htm*

'5 Reasons Cancer and Sugar are Best Friends': *http://beatcancer.org/2014/03/5-reasons-cancer-and-sugar-are-best-friends/*

But the important point is here that as raw foods contain anti-cancer compounds, as most of them alkalize the body so they can limit cancerous cells, while refined sugar and cooked starch cannot, and they even speed up cancer growth.

The QR codes related to links above (endnote number 30) in sequence (from left):

[31] Cancer cells are anaerobic cells.

[32] Actually they are there in response to oxygen deprivation. They are primitive cells that can save us if we will listen.

[33] However this opinion maybe not true. Everything the body does has a purpose. There is always a reason if we understand the body. The body's main goal is to create a constant balance – homeostasis, not to blindly fill in blank spots. Cancer cells are not connected to the body's communication system at all and grow at will as long as they have the fuel they need – glucose for energy and fructose to multiply rapidly.

[34] Page 11 of the mentioned book (Cancer Cells, by Edmund Vincent Cowdry)

[35] Page 15 of the mentioned book (Cancer Cells, by Edmund Vincent Cowdry)

[36] Page 333 of the mentioned book (Cancer Cells, by Edmund Vincent Cowdry)

[37] Page 39 of the mentioned book (Cancer Cells, by Edmund Vincent Cowdry)

[38] Page 152 of the mentioned book (Cancer Cells, by Edmund Vincent Cowdry)

[39] Page 101 and 102 of the mentioned book (Cancer Cells, by Edmund Vincent Cowdry)

[40] Page 151 and 152 of the mentioned book (Cancer Cells, by Edmund Vincent Cowdry)

[41] Page 220 of the mentioned book (Cancer Cells, by Edmund Vincent Cowdry)

[42] *http://www.cancer.gov/*

[43] Adopted from:

Biographical Sketch: Otto Heinrich Warburg, PhD, MD:
http://www.ncbi.nlm.nih.gov/pmc/articles/PMC2947689/

The Prime Cause and Prevention of Cancer: *http://www.healingcancernaturally.com/warburgcancer-cause-prevention.html*

The QR codes related to links above in sequence (from left):

[44] *http://andrealambert.net/about-andrea/*

[45] Lifestyle Without Cancer_ by Andrea Lambert_ Page 4.

[46] Same as the previous reference_ page 5.

[47] Same as the previous reference_ page 8.

[48] Same as the previous reference_ pages 18 and 19.

[49] Read the article '*How Much Protein Does a Human Body Need Daily to Maintain Muscle?*':
http://www.livestrong.com/article/523623-how-much-protein-does-a-human-body-need-daily-to-maintain-muscle/

[50] Read the articles:
'Putting Meat Back in Its Place' New York Times:
http://www.nytimes.com/2008/06/11/dining/11mini.html?pagewanted=all&_r=0

'Protein Content of Green Vegetables compared to Meat?':
https://www.drfuhrman.com/faq/question.aspx?sid=16&qindex=9

[51] Read the article: '*Too much protein could lead to early death, study says*' on The Washington Post:
http://www.washingtonpost.com/national/health-science/too-much-protein-could-lead-to-early-death-study-says/2014/03/04/0af0603e-a3b5-11e3-8466-d34c451760b9_story.html

The QR codes related to 49-51 in sequence at next page(from left):

[52] 'Protein and the Athlete – How Much Do You Need?':
http://www.eatright.org/Public/content.aspx?id=6442477918

[53] '*Healthy or not: the truth about athletes' diets*' on The Free Press_ the official student newspaper of the University of Southern Maine: *http://usmfreepress.org/2014/03/03/healthy-or-not-the-truth-about-athletes-diets/*

The QR codes related to 52-53 in sequence (from left):

[54] See the article '*Mad Cow Disease Fast Facts*' by CNN Library:
http://www.cnn.com/2013/07/02/health/mad-cow-disease-fast-facts/

[55] Read the articles:
'5 Surprising Health Benefits of Eating Less Meat': *http://beyondmeat.com/5-surprising-health-benefits-of-eating-less-meat/*

'A Vegetarian Diet Can Help With Impotence':
http://www.peta.org/living/food/impotence/?search=impotence

[56] Read '*The composition of human milk*' on the National Institutes of Health:
http://www.ncbi.nlm.nih.gov/pubmed/392766

And the article: ' *A comparison between human milk and cow's milk*':
http://www.vegetarian.org.uk/campaigns/whitelies/wlreport05.shtml

The QR codes related to 55-56 in sequence (from left):

[57] See '*Protein Content of Fruits*' on whole food catalog:
http://wholefoodcatalog.info/nutrient/protein/fruits/

[58] ' The Effects of Not Enough Protein in the Diet': *http://www.livestrong.com/article/256074-the-effects-of-not-enough-protein-in-the-diet/*

[59] *http://www.ncbi.nlm.nih.gov/pmc/articles/PMC3854817/*

[60] For more information, read the article '*Food - Raw Versus Cooked*':
http://jonbarron.org/article/food-raw-versus-cooked#.U-T27vmSxBE

The QR codes related to 57-60 in sequence in next page (from left):

[61] Read the article '*Your body recycling itself -- captured on film*' on ScienceDaily :
http://www.sciencedaily.com/releases/2010/09/100913093038.htm

[62] 'Fasting In Nature': *http://www.rawfoodexplained.com/introduction-to-fasting/fasting-in-nature.html*

The QR codes related to 61-62 in sequence (from left):

[63] Read the articles: '*High-protein diet 'as bad for health as smoking'* on Telegraph: *http://www.telegraph.co.uk/science/science-news/10676877/High-protein-diet-as-bad-for-health-as-smoking.html*

'Diets high in meat, eggs and dairy could be as harmful to health as smoking': *http://www.theguardian.com/science/2014/mar/04/animal-protein-diets-smoking-meat-eggs-dairy*

'Signs & Symptoms of Too Much Protein in the Diet': *http://www.livestrong.com/article/253065-signs-symptoms-of-too-much-protein-in-the-diet/*

The QR codes related to links above in sequence (from left):

[64] 'Protein From Animal Products is More Harmful Than From Plants': *http://www.collective-evolution.com/2011/12/16/the-protein-myth-eat-your-meat/*

[65] Adopted from: *http://michaelbluejay.com/veg/protein.html*

[66] Quoted from: *http://www.diseaseproof.com/archives/diet-myths-complementary-protein-myth-wont-go-away.html*

[67] 'Plant Foods Have a Complete Amino Acid Composition': *http://circ.ahajournals.org/content/105/25/e197.full*

The QR codes related to 64-67 in sequence in next page(from left):

[68] More information, read the article '*Debunking the milk myth*':
http://saveourbones.com/osteoporosis-milk-myth/

[69] Read the article '*For Good Bone Health, Break Your Dairy Addiction*' on PETA:
http://prime.peta.org/2012/04/addiction

[70] A very good resource for more information about bone health is the Book 'The Calcium Lie' by Dr. Robert Thompson: *http://www.CalciumLie.com/*

[71] For more information, read the article ' *Dangers of Pasteurization and Homogenization*':
http://preventdisease.com/news/10/111810_dangers_pasteurization_homogenization.shtml

The QR codes related to 68-71 in sequence (from left):

[72] *http://www.tcolincampbell.org/*

[73] *www.notmilk.com*

[74] For more information about these dangers, read '*Raw Milk Questions and Answers*' in Center for Disease Control and Prevention:
http://www.cdc.gov/foodsafety/rawmilk/raw-milk-questions-and-answers.html

[75] More information in the article '*Lactic Acid Found To Fuel Tumors*' on Science Daily:
http://www.sciencedaily.com/releases/2008/11/081120171325.htm

[76] Resource: '*Battling Bad Breath*' on the Dr. OZ show:
http://www.doctoroz.com/blog/jonathan-b-levine-dmd/battling-bad-breath

[77] Resource: '*Milk causes bad breath in several ways*':
http://www.therabreath.com/articles/blog/oral-care-tips-and-advice/milk-causes-bad-breath-in-several-ways-3565.asp

The QR codes related to 74-77 in sequence in next page (from left):

[78] Resource: *'Bad Breath Lifestyle Tips'*:
http://www.badbreath.com.au/article/lifestyle-tips-bad-breath.html

[79] You can access all archives of Science magazine on: *http://www.sciencemag.org/*

[80] For more information, go to the vegetarian starter kit on PCRM:
http://www.pcrm.org/health/diets/vsk/vegetarian-starter-kit-calcium

and also read the Article 'Calcium and Strong Bones' on PCRM:
http://www.pcrm.org/health/health-topics/calcium-and-strong-bones

The QR codes related to 78-80 in sequence (from left):

[81] *'Benefits of Sunlight: A Bright Spot for Human Health'* from the National Institutes of Health:
http://www.ncbi.nlm.nih.gov/pmc/articles/PMC2290997/

[82] *'Vitamin D: Fact Sheet for Health Professionals'*_ National Institutes of Health:
http://ods.od.nih.gov/factsheets/VitaminD-HealthProfessional/#en1

[83] *'Vitamin D: Fact Sheet for Health Professionals'*_ National Institutes of Health:
http://ods.od.nih.gov/factsheets/VitaminD-HealthProfessional/#en1

[84] ' *Sunlight and vitamin D for bone health and prevention of autoimmune diseases, cancers, and cardiovascular disease*' by Michael F. Holick on American Society for Clinical nutrition: *http://ajcn.nutrition.org/content/80/6/1678S.full*

The QR codes related to 81-84 in sequence (from left):

[85] Quoted from '*Benefits of Sunlight: A Bright Spot for Human Health*' from the National Institutes of Health: *http://www.ncbi.nlm.nih.gov/pmc/articles/PMC2290997/*

[86] Quoted form the article '*How does a lack of sun affect us*' on Discovery: *http://curiosity.discovery.com/question/affects-of-lack-of-sun*

[87] *http://www.doctoroz.com/videos/your-sunscreen-might-be-poisoning-you*

The QR codes related to 85-87 in sequence (from left):

[88] '*Ask the Expert: Omega-3 Fatty Acids*' from The Nutrition Source, Harvard School of Public Health: *http://www.hsph.harvard.edu/nutritionsource/omega-3/*

[89] For more information, see:

Non-Fish Sources of Omega 3 : *http://www.livestrong.com/article/287214-non-fish-sources-of-omega-3/*

Omega-3 Fatty Acids and Antioxidants in Edible Wild Plants: *http://www.scielo.cl/pdf/bres/v37n2/art13.pdf*

This useful article about essential fatty acids: *http://aliverawfoods.com/faqs/essential-fatty-acids/*

The QR codes related to 88-89 in sequence (from left, here and next page):

[90] Read the article 'The importance of the ratio of omega-6/omega-3 essential fatty acids' from the National Institutes of Health : *http://www.ncbi.nlm.nih.gov/pubmed/12442909*

[91] *'Omega-6 fatty acids'* on the University of Maryland Medical System : *http://umm.edu/health/medical/altmed/supplement/omega6-fatty-acids*

[92] *'Does Smoking Deplete B12 ?'*: *http://vitamins.lovetoknow.com/Does_Smoking_Deplete_B12*

[93] Find out more about Dr. Zarin Azar on PCRM: *http://www.pcrm.org/good-medicine/2004/winter/physician-profile-zarin-azar-md*

The QR codes related to 90-93 in sequence (from left):

[94] The Article *'Getting Enough B12?'*: *http://enews.tufts.edu/stories/1263/2001/09/10/GettingEnoughB12*

[95] References and Resources:
'Fit for Life' by Diamond, H. and M., 1987
'Nutrition and Athletic Performance' by Dr. Douglas Graham, 1999
'Human Anatomy and Physiology' by Elaine N. Marieb – 1999
Rethinking B12 article by Dr V. V. Vetrano
'The Vitamin B12 Issue' by Dr. Gina Shaw: *http://www.vibrancyuk.com/B12.html*
The Article: *'Vitamin B12 Deficiency—the Meat-eaters' Last Stand'* in Dr. John McDougall's website: *http://www.drmcdougall.com/misc/2007nl/nov/071100.htm*

The QR codes related to links above in sequence at next page (from left):

[96] For more information, you can refer to the article '*Controversy in the Measurement of Vitamin B12 Levels*':
http://www.dsm.com/campaigns/talkingnutrition/en_US/talkingnutrition-dsm-com/2013/09/vitamin-B12-measurement-controversy-HCY2013.html

[97] Quoted from the article '*Why don't the teeth of animals decay though they never brush their teeth?*':
http://timesofindia.indiatimes.com/home/stoi/Why-dont-the-teeth-of-animals-decay-though-they-never-brush-their-teeth/articleshow/4739033.cms

[98] For more and complete details, read the article '*Dr. Herbert Shelton on the true causes of tooth decay*': *http://www.healingteethnaturally.com/dr-herbert-shelton-real-reasons-tooth-decay.html*

[99] Adopted from the article '*The Real Cause of Tooth Decay (and How to Stop it Naturally)*':
http://www.smallfootprintfamily.com/how-to-stop-tooth-decay

The QR codes related to 96-99 in sequence (from left):

[100] '*The Alkaline Diet: Is There Evidence That an Alkaline pH Diet Benefits Health?*' published on U.S. national library of medicine: *http://www.ncbi.nlm.nih.gov/pmc/articles/PMC3195546/*
'Acid Vs. Alkaline: The Science Behind Balancing Your pH': *http://vidyacleanse.com/2013/03/acid-vs-alkaline-the-science-behind-balancing-your-ph/*

[101] See '*Definition of Poison*': *http://www.medterms.com/script/main/art.asp?articlekey=11890*

[102] Even some scientific studies show that it is a cancer suppressor, for example this article from the Journal of Natural Products: *http://pubs.acs.org/doi/abs/10.1021/np000592z?journalCode=jnprdf*

The QR codes related to 100-102 in sequence at next page (from left):

[103] For more information read the article '*When a little poison is good for you*' from the New Scientist: *http://www.newscientist.com/article/mg19926681.700-when-a-little-poison-is-good-for-you.html*

This article with the same title as above, which debunked some misconceptions in this regard: *http://articles.mercola.com/sites/articles/archive/2008/08/30/when-a-little-poison-is-good-for-you.aspx*

An article in Fortune Magazine entitles '*A Little Poison Can Be Good For You: The received wisdom about toxins and radiation may be all wet.*': *http://archive.fortune.com/magazines/fortune/fortune_archive/2003/06/09/343948/index.htm*

[104] See the article '*How bad is junk food for your DNA*': *http://wakeup-world.com/2012/07/22/how-bad-is-junk-food-for-your-dna/*

The QR codes related to 103-104 in sequence (from left):

[105] See the article '*Diet and cancer: the evidence*' in Cancer Research UK: *http://www.cancerresearchuk.org/cancer-info/healthyliving/dietandhealthyeating/howdoweknow/diet-and-cancer-the-evidence*

[106] For more information, you can see here: *http://www.wisegeek.com/what-is-solanine.htm*

[107] See the article '*How Lectin In Undercooked Red Beans And Rice Causes Food Poisoning*' from Medical News Today: *http://www.medicalnewstoday.com/releases/78478.php*

Also the article '*Hemagglutinin and Food Poisoning from Beans*' in Chemistry.About.com explains that why it's not safe to eat raw beans:
 http://chemistry.about.com/b/2014/02/05/hemagglutinin-and-food-poisoning-from-beans.htm

The QR codes related to 105-107 in sequence (from left):

[108] Read the articles:

'Tea Side Effects: Top 10 Bad Effects Of Tea On health': *http://www.healthmw.com/20/02/2012/mens-health/tea-side-effects-top-10-bad-effects-of-tea-on-health-49.html*

'Could Tea Be Bad For You? 5 Tea Ingredients That Are Harming Your Health': *http://www.medicaldaily.com/could-tea-be-bad-you-5-tea-ingredients-are-harming-your-health-253445*

'Is your coffee habit killing you or saving your life?': *http://www.today.com/health/your-coffee-habit-killing-you-or-saving-your-life-2D11603303*

[109] See the article 'Soy Controversy and The Effects of Soy Consumption' by Dr. Joseph Mercola: *http://articles.mercola.com/sites/articles/archive/2010/10/13/soy-controversy-and-health-effects.aspx*

The QR codes related to 108-109 in sequence (from left):

[110] See the Article '*Soy and the Thyroid – A Look at the Controversy*' :
http://thyroid.about.com/cs/soyinfo/a/soy.htm

[111] Read the article '*AFLATOXINS : Occurrence and Health Risks*' from Cornell University-college of Agriculture and Life Sciences: *http://www.ansci.cornell.edu/plants/toxicagents/aflatoxin/aflatoxin.html*

[112] See the article: '*Cancer biologists find DNA-damaging toxins in common plant-based foods*' on Science Daily Magazine: *http://www.sciencedaily.com/releases/2013/03/130327163302.htm*

The QR codes related to 110-112 in sequence (from left):

[113] '*Using natural laws in healthy eating*' (the book is in Persian and this is a translation of its Persian title by me)_ by Dr. Abdolhossein Navab_ Page 194

[114] '*Caffeine for Your Health — Too Good to Be True?*':
http://www.aarp.org/health/healthy-living/info-10-2013/coffee-for-health.html

[115] Read the articles:
'Apples: the healthier alternative to coffee': *http://www.personal.psu.edu/afr3/blogs/siowfa12/2012/09/apples-wake-you-awake-more-than-coffee-does.html*

'Does Eating an Apple in the Morning Wake You Up Better Than Drinking a Cup of Coffee?':
http://www.livestrong.com/article/547850-does-eating-an-apple-in-the-morning-wake-you-up-better-than-drinking-a-cup-of-cofee/

The QR codes related to 114-115 in sequence in next page (from left):

[116] If you want to enjoy recipes, I only recommend **Low Fat Vegan/Raw Vegan** recipes which are **Gluten-free** also **Salt-free.**

[117] Adopted from:
http://www.beautifulonraw.com/raw-food-blog/raw-food-lifestyle/why-you-need-to-soak-your-nuts/

[118] Information from: *http://www.veggiewave.com/*

[119] *http://www.cancer.org/cancer/cancercauses/othercarcinogens/athome/acrylamide*

[120] '*New understanding of gluten sensitivity*' by Volta U & De Giorgio R.
(*http://www.ncbi.nlm.nih.gov/pubmed/22371218*) Nat Rev Gastroenterol Hepatol. 2012; Advance Online Publication: doi:10.1038/nrgastro.2012.15.

The QR codes related to 117-120 in sequence (from left):

[121] For more information, read the article "Symptoms of Gluten Intolerance are very common": *http://www.easy-immune-health.com/Symptoms-of-Gluten-Intolerance.html*

[122] From the article '*When Wheat Muffins Turn to The Dark Side: on Gluten and Your Diet*': *http://www.scq.ubc.ca/when-wheat-muffins-turn-to-the-dark-side-on-gluten-and-your-diet/*

[123] 'Warning: Fluoride in Drinking Water Is Damaging Your Bones, Brain, Kidneys, and Thyroid': *http://articles.mercola.com/sites/articles/archive/2010/07/01/paul-connett-interview.aspx*

The QR codes related to 121-123 in sequence (from left):

[124] '50 REASONS TO OPPOSE FLUORIDATION': *http://fluoridealert.org/articles/50-reasons/*

'ADA study confirms dangers of fluoridated water, especially for babies': *http://www.naturalnews.com/030123_fluoride_babies.html*

[125] 'The Health Dangers of Table Salt': *http://www.globalhealingcenter.com/natural-health/dangers-of-salt/*

The QR codes related to 124-125 in sequence (from left):

[126] References related to Iodine:

'Iodine fact sheet for health professionals': *http://ods.od.nih.gov/factsheets/Iodine-HealthProfessional/*

'Iodine in diet': *http://www.nlm.nih.gov/medlineplus/ency/article/002421.htm*

'Iodine_ fact sheet for consumers': *http://ods.od.nih.gov/factsheets/Iodine-Consumer/*

About Iodine supplementation and side effects:
http://www.nlm.nih.gov/medlineplus/druginfo/natural/35.html

'Dietary Iodine': *http://www.30bananasaday.com/profiles/blogs/dietary-iodine*

The QR codes related to links above (endnote number 126) in sequence (from left):

[127] The Dead Sea is one of the world's saltiest bodies of water, named because its salinity makes it too harsh an environment for any animals to flourish.

[128] The complete interview in Raw Vegan Radio:
http://www.rawveganradio.com/the-gerson-way-with-charlotte-gerson/

[129] Luke RG. Transactions of the American Clinical and Climatological Association, Vol. 118, 2007. President's Address: Salt – too much of a good thing?

[130] Tuomilehto J et al. Urinary sodium excretion and cardiovascular mortality in Finland: a prospective study. Lancet 2001;357:848-851

[131] American Society of Nephrology: *http://asn-online.org*

[132] H, R., and Y. Suyama. 1996. Sodium excretion in relation to calcium and hydroxyproline excretion in a healthy Japanese population. Am. J. Clin. Nutr. 63 (5): 735-40.

[133] Yano K et al. Serum Cholesterol and Hemorrhagic Stroke in the Honolulu Heart Program. Stroke 1989;20(11):1460-1465

[134] Tsugane S, Sasazuki S. Diet and the risk of gastric cancer. Gastric Cancer 2007;10(2):75-83

[135] Burney P. A diet rich in sodium may potentiate asthma. Epidemiologic evidence for a new hypothesis. Chest 1987;91 (2 Suppl):143s-148s

[136] Other useful references about salt:

Fatal Poisoning From Salt Used as an Emetic, Jorge Barer, MD; L. Leighton Hill, MD; Reba M. Hill, MD; Waldo M. Martinez, MD _ Am J Dis Child. 1973:
http://archpedi.jamanetwork.com/article.aspx?articleid=505041

'Salt: More than High Blood Pressure' _ Dr. Joel Fuhrman:
https://www.drfuhrman.com/library/salt_more_than_high_blood_pressure.aspx

'Should I avoid salt?' _ Dr. Joel Fuhrman:
https://www.drfuhrman.com/faq/question.aspx?sid=16&qindex=1

[137] 'Overview of Salt Toxicity':
http://www.merckmanuals.com/vet/toxicology/salt_toxicity/overview_of_salt_toxicity.html

The QR codes related to 136-137 in sequence (from left):

[138] 'Will Sodium Deficiency Correct Itself?':
http://healthyeating.sfgate.com/sodium-deficiency-correct-itself-6770.html

[139] 'Signs of Sodium Deficiency': http://www.livestrong.com/article/417785-signs-of-sodium-deficiency/

[140] For more information about Salicornia herb, its benefits and scientific research about it, read the article *'Spherical Granule Production from Micronized Saltwort (Salicornia herbacea) Powder as Salt Substitute'* featured on the National Institute of Health's website :
http://www.ncbi.nlm.nih.gov/pmc/articles/PMC3867153/

And also it's PDF version:
http://www.ncbi.nlm.nih.gov/pmc/articles/PMC3867153/pdf/pnf_2013_v18n1_60.pdf

The QR codes related to 138-140 in sequence in next page (from left):

[141] Recommended articles for more information:
'Fruits – Mighty Good For Your Health':
http://breastcancer.about.com/od/cancerfightingfoods/a/fruits_benefits.htm

'*Phenolic Phytochemicals in Fruits and Vegetables are Linked to Health Benefits*' by Dr. Kalidas Shetty_ University of Massachusetts Amherst:
http://www.newenglandvfc.org/pdf_proceedings/2009/ppfvlhb.pdf

'*Health benefits of fruit and vegetables are from additive and synergistic combinations of phytochemicals*' from the American Society for Clinical Nutrition:
http://ajcn.nutrition.org/content/78/3/517S.full

'*Phenol Antioxidant Quantity and Quality in Foods: Fruits*' from the American Chemical Society:
http://pubs.acs.org/doi/abs/10.1021/jf0009293

Phenolic Acid -- Plant Antioxidant: *http://nutrition.about.com/od/nutrition101/a/Phenolic-Acids.htm*

[142] Read the article '*The Dangers of Pesticides*': *http://www.nature.com/scitable/blog/green-science/the_dangers_of_pesticides*

[143] Read the complete news with the title '*Pesticide, fertilizer mixes linked to range of health problems*' : *http://www.news.wisc.edu/290*

[144] See the Article '*Removing Pesticides from Fruits and Vegetables*' at Centre for Science and Environment: *http://www.cseindia.org/content/removing-pesticides-fruits-and-vegetables*

The QR codes related to 141-144 in sequence (from left, here and next page):

[145] Read the article: "Chronic intake of potato chips in humans increases the production of reactive oxygen radicals by leukocytes and increases plasma C-reactive protein: a pilot study" from the American Society for nutrition: *http://ajcn.nutrition.org/content/89/3/773.full*

[146] The complete article "Position of the American Dietetic Association: Vegetarian Diets"_PDF version: *http://www.eatright.org/WorkArea/linkit.aspx?LinkIdentifier=id&ItemID=8417*

The summary online version of the mentioned article: *http://www.ncbi.nlm.nih.gov/pubmed/19562864*

[147] The quoted article is also published on Science Daily: *http://www.sciencedaily.com/releases/2009/07/090701103002.htm*

The QR codes related to 145-147 in sequence (from left):

[148] Link to the mentioned article published by the National Institutes of Health: *http://www.ncbi.nlm.nih.gov/pubmed/15702597*

"[149] Read the article 'Hypnosis/local anesthesia combination during surgery helps patients, reduces hospital stays, study finds' on Science Daily: *http://www.sciencedaily.com/releases/2011/06/110613012819.htm*

The QR codes related to 148-149 in sequence at next page(from left):

[150] Some articles covering this subject:

'Diagnostic Errors More Common, Costly And Harmful Than Treatment Mistakes':
http://www.hopkinsmedicine.org/news/media/releases/diagnostic_errors_more_common_costly_and_h armful_than_treatment_mistakes

'Diagnostic Errors Are the Most Common Type of Medical Mistake':
http://healthland.time.com/2013/04/24/diagnostic-errors-are-more-common-and-harmful-for-patients/

'Testing Mistakes at the Family Doctor':
http://well.blogs.nytimes.com/2008/08/14/testing-mistakes-at-the-family-doctor/?_php=true&_type=blogs&_r=0

'More Treatment, More Mistakes':
http://www.nytimes.com/2012/08/01/opinion/more-treatment-more-mistakes.html

The QR codes related to links above (number 150) in sequence (from left):

[151] Biochemistry. 5th edition._ Berg JM, Tymoczko JL, Stryer L._ Section 30.2Each Organ Has a Unique Metabolic Profile: *http://www.ncbi.nlm.nih.gov/books/NBK22436/*

[152] Link to the mentioned article: *http://www.fredericpatenaude.com/blog/?p=283*

[153] '15 Foods to Improve Your Memory Naturally and Boost Brain Power':
http://www.sunwarrior.com/news/brain-foods/

[154] "Why Eat Raw?":
http://www.nursezone.com/Nursing-News-Events/devices-and-technology.aspx?articleID=11566

The QR codes related to 151-154 in sequence at next page (from left):

[155] For example:

"Raw Foods and Nutrition to Heal Damaged Tissues from an Accident":
http://www.blanelaw.com/practice_areas/san-diego-ca-raw-foods.cfm

'An Incredible Recovery from Brain Surgery with Organic & Raw Vegan Food: 28-Day Body & Soul Detox' video on Youtube: *http://www.youtube.com/watch?v=iwdsu8Loh4Y*

[156] Read Tanya's full story on her website: *http://betterraw.com/about*

[157] '*Animal Intelligence Under-rated By Humans, Researchers Say*' :
http://www.natureworldnews.com/articles/5194/20131205/humans-smarter-animals-researchers.htm

The QR codes related to 155-157 in sequence (from left):

[158] *http://ancienthistory.about.com/cs/grecoromanmyth1/a/hesiodagesofman.htm*

[159] As an example, read the article 'China's Soils Ruined by Overuse of Chemical Fertilizers':
http://www.i-sis.org.uk/chinasSoilRuined.php

The QR codes related to 158-159 in sequence at next page (from left):

[160] More scientific details about the importance of alkalizing the body are explained in the book '*The Meaning of True Health*' by Dr. Chang Jia Rui.

[161] *http://www.enviroingenuity.com/articles/synthetic-vs-organic-fertilizers.html*

[162] 'Will Organic Food Fail to Feed the World?':
http://www.scientificamerican.com/article/organic-farming-yields-and-feeding-the-world-under-climate-change/

'Can organic food feed the world? New study sheds light on debate over organic vs. conventional agriculture' :*http://www.sciencedaily.com/releases/2012/04/120425140114.htm*

'Can Organic Farming Feed Us All?' : *http://www.worldwatch.org/node/4060*

The QR codes related to 161-162 in sequence (from left):

[163] 'Feeding the future: How organic farming can help feed the world':
http://www.soilassociation.org/motherearth/viewarticle/articleid/3457/feeding-the-future-how-organic-farming-can-help-feed-the-world

'Organic Can Feed the World':
http://www.theatlantic.com/health/archive/2011/12/organic-can-feed-the-world/249348/

[164] *http://www.fao.org/organicag/oa-faq/oa-faq7/en/*

[165] Adopted from the article '*The Clean 15: Foods You Don't Have to Buy Organic*':
http://www.goodhousekeeping.com/recipes/healthy/Save-on-Sustainable-Gallery-44032808#slide-1

The QR codes related to 163-165 in sequence at next page (from left):

[166] *http://health.ninemsn.com.au/whats-good-for-you/*

[167] Article link: *http://www.theguardian.com/lifeandstyle/2010/jul/18/vegetarianism-save-planet-environment*

[168] Article link: http://www.care2.com/causes/the-true-cost-of-meat-demystifying-agricultural-subsidies.html

[169] Read the complete article '*10 Things I Wish All Americans Knew About The Meat and Dairy Industries*' on the official website of MEATONOMICS: *http://meatonomics.com/2013/09/28/10-things-i-wish-all-americans-knew-about-the-meat-dairy-industries/*

The QR codes related to 166-169 in sequence in next page(from left):

[170] The article "Agricultural Policies Versus Health Policies" from PCRM: *http://pcrm.org/health/reports/agriculture-and-health-policies-ag-versus-health*

[171] A good resource for more information: '*Some Economic Benefits and Costs of Vegetarianism*' _Jayson L. Lusk and F. Bailey Norwood _ available for download from the University of Minnesota: *http://ageconsearch.umn.edu/bitstream/55529/2/lusk%20-%20current.pdf*

[172] For more information: *http://intellectualyst.com/be-angry-the-government-subsidies-poor-health/*

And see the article from the New York Times:
http://economix.blogs.nytimes.com/2010/03/09/why-a-big-mac-costs-less-than-a-salad/

The QR codes related to 170-172 in sequence (from left):

[173] Reference: The main article '*Climate benefits of changing diet*' on PBL Netherlands Environmental Assessment Agency: *http://www.pbl.nl/en/publications/2009/Climate-benefits-of-changing-diet*

[174] Quoted from: *www.veganoutreach.org*

[175] Note: The term 'livestock' refers to all farmed animals, including pigs, birds raised for meat, egg-laying hens, and dairy cows.

[176] 'Livestock a major threat to environment':
http://www.fao.org/newsroom/en/news/2006/1000448/index.html

[177] *http://www.epa.gov/region9/animalwaste/problem.html*

[178] '*Corporate Welfare: The Empire Of The Pigs*'_ TIME, 30 November 1998:
http://www.time.com/time/magazine/article/0,9171,989675,00.html

[179] For more information on the harmful effects of meat eating on environment see the article by Lacey Gaechter found at Vegan Outreach: *http://www.veganoutreach.org/whyvegan/gaechter.html*

The QR codes related to 176-179 in sequence (from left, at next page):

[180] *http://www.worldwatch.org/files/pdf/Livestock%20and%20Climate%20Change.pdf*

[181] From the article '*Study claims meat creates half of all greenhouse gases*' in The Independent: *http://www.independent.co.uk/environment/climate-change/study-claims-meat-creates-half-of-all-greenhouse-gases-1812909.html*

[182] See the article '*Are cows the cause of global warming?*': *http://timeforchange.org/are-cows-cause-of-global-warming-meat-methane-CO2*

[183] See the article '*Methane impact on global warming 'much greater than thought*': *http://www.telegraph.co.uk/earth/earthnews/6466890/Methane-impact-on-global-warming-much-greater-than-thought.html*

The QR codes related to 180-183 in sequence (from left):

[184] For more information:

'Evaluating the environmental impact of various dietary patterns combined with different food production systems': *http://www.nature.com/ejcn/journal/v61/n2/full/1602522a.html*

'*Dietary choices and greenhouse gas emissions*' – assessment of impact of vegetarian and organic options at national scale: *http://inderscience.metapress.com/content/mg413q602lr84803/*

'*The Economic and Taste Benefits of a Vegetarian Diet*' _by Gary Null, PhD, and Martin Feldman, MD : *http://www.townsendletter.com/Oct2011/vege1011.html*

[185] The article '*Climate benefits of changing diet*':
http://www.pbl.nl/en/publications/2009/Climate-benefits-of-changing-diet

The QR codes related to 184-185 in sequence (from left):

[186] From the article '*10 ways vegetarianism can help save the planet*' published in The Guardian:
http://www.theguardian.com/lifeandstyle/2010/jul/18/vegetarianism-save-planet-environment

[187] See the article '*What if Everyone in the World Became a Vegetarian?*' in Slate Online Magazine:
http://www.slate.com/articles/health_and_science/feed_the_world/2014/05/meat_eating_and_climate_change_vegetarians_impact_on_the_economy_antibiotics.html

[188] See the article '*U.S. Meat Production*' on Oregon Physicians for Social Responsibility :
http://www.psr.org/chapters/oregon/safe-food/industrial-meat-system.html

[189] The article '*Plants Can Benefit from Herbivory: Stimulatory Effects of Sheep Saliva on Growth of Leymus chinensis*' on Plos One:
http://www.plosone.org/article/info%3Adoi%2F10.1371%2Fjournal.pone.0029259

The QR codes related to 186-189 in sequence (from left, here and next page):

[190] The complete article '*Large herbivores can play critical role in maintaining ecosystem health*' on Stanford University news website: *http://news.stanford.edu/news/2007/january17/pringle-011707.html*

[191] For more information, See also:

'*The Pain Behind Foie Gras*':
http://www.peta.org/issues/animals-used-for-food/animals-used-food-factsheets/pain-behind-foie-gras/

'How Is Foie Gras Particularly Cruel to Animals?':
http://animalrights.about.com/od/FactoryFarming/a/Foie-Gras.htm

Foie Gras Controversy on Wikipedia: *http://en.wikipedia.org/wiki/Foie_gras_controversy*

The QR codes related to 190-191 in sequence (from left):

[192] For example: '*Meat and cheese may be as bad for you as smoking*':
http://www.sciencedaily.com/releases/2014/03/140304125639.htm

[193] This research article is also useful:

Lowe, Brian M.; Ginsberg, Caryn F. : '*Animal Rights as a Post-Citizenship Movement*' from Society and Animals, Volume 10, Number 2, 2002 , pp. 203-215(13):
http://dx.doi.org/10.1163/156853002320292345

[194] See the article *'Toxins in Our Honey?'* from the Centre for Food Safety of Hong Kong: *http://www.cfs.gov.hk/english/multimedia/multimedia_pub/multimedia_pub_fsf_89_02.html*

[195] See the article *'Side Effects of Eating Too Much Honey'* at Live Strong: *http://www.livestrong.com/article/410468-side-effects-of-eating-too-much-honey/*

The QR codes related to 193-195 in sequence (from left, at next page):

[196] 'Entomologists: "Stop feeding corn syrup to honeybees." Duh.': *http://grist.org/news/entomologists-stop-feeding-corn-syrup-to-honeybees-duh/*

[197] 'Feeding Refined Sugar to Honey Bees': *http://www.motherearthnews.com/homesteading-and-livestock/feeding-refined-sugar-to-honey-bees.aspx*

[198] More information about honey and honeybees: *http://www.vegetus.org/honey/honey.htm*

The QR codes related to 196-198 in sequence (from left):

[199] The book *'Language of Foods'* (in Persian) by Dr. Ghiassedin Jazayeri

[200] 'How can you make chickens lay more eggs?': *http://www.answers.com/Q/How_can_you_make_chickens_lay_more_eggs*

[201] 'Happy Cows: Behind the Myth': *http://www.humanemyth.org/happycows.htm*

[202] See the article: *'Study links bee decline to cell phones'* on CNN: *http://www.cnn.com/2010/WORLD/europe/06/30/bee.decline.mobile.phones/*

The QR codes related to 201-202 in sequence in next page(from left):

[203] See his website: *www.scottjurek.com*

[204] Examples of more vegan athletes in: *http://www.bestveganguide.com/vegan-athletes.html*

Printed in Great Britain
by Amazon.co.uk, Ltd.,
Marston Gate.